Questions & Answers About Diseases of the Pancreas

Timothy B. Gardner, MD
Director, Pancreatic Disorders
Section of Gastroenterology and Hepatology
Dartmouth-Hitchcock Medical Center
Lebanon, NH

Andrew S. Warner, MD
Chairman, Department of Gastroenterology
Lahey Clinic
Burlington, MA

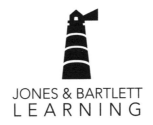

JONES & BARTLETT
L E A R N I N G

World Headquarters
Jones & Bartlett Learning
5 Wall Street
Burlington, MA 01803
info@jblearning.com
www.jblearning.com

Jones & Bartlett Learning books and products are available through most bookstores and online booksellers. To contact Jones & Bartlett Learning directly, call 800-832-0034, fax 978-443-8000, or visit our website, www.jblearning.com.

Substantial discounts on bulk quantities of Jones & Bartlett Learning publications are available to corporations, professional associations, and other qualified organizations. For details and specific discount information, contact the special sales department at Jones & Bartlett Learning via the above contact information or send an email to specialsales@jblearning.com.

The authors, editor, and publisher have made every effort to provide accurate information. However, they are not responsible for errors, omissions, or for any outcomes related to the use of the contents of this book and take no responsibility for the use of the products and procedures described. Treatments and side effects described in this book may not be applicable to all people; likewise, some people may require a dose or experience a side effect that is not described herein. Drugs and medical devices are discussed that may have limited availability controlled by the Food and Drug Administration (FDA) for use only in a research study or clinical trial. Research, clinical practice, and government regulations often change the accepted standard in this field. When consideration is being given to use of any drug in the clinical setting, the healthcare provider or reader is responsible for determining FDA status of the drug, reading the package insert, and reviewing prescribing information for the most up-to-date recommendations on dose, precautions, and contraindications, and determining the appropriate usage for the product. This is especially important in the case of drugs that are new or seldom used.

Production Credits
Executive Publisher: Christopher Davis
Managing Editor, Custom Projects: Kathy Richardson
Production Assistant: Leia Poritz
Manufacturing and Inventory Control Supervisor: Amy Bacus
Composition: Abella Publishing Services

Cover Design: Carolyn Downer
Cover Images: Top left photo: © Rubberball Productions;
        Top right photo: © Biljana Kumer/ShutterStock, Inc.;
        Bottom photo: © Digital Vision/Getty Images
Printing and Binding: Malloy, Inc.
Cover Printing: Malloy, Inc.

Unless otherwise indicated, all photographs and illustrations are under copyright of Jones & Bartlett Learning.

ISBN: 978-1-4496-7032-0

6048

Printed in the United States of America
16 15 14 13 12   10 9 8 7 6 5 4 3 2 1

This is dedicated to our patients and our families.

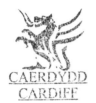

Contents

Disorders of the pancreas, from pancreatitis to pancreatic cancer, affect millions of patients and their families worldwide. Surprisingly, despite so many people having these diseases, there is little information available to help deal with these serious conditions. We frequently heard from our patients that there just was not a simple, yet informative, guide for updated information on disorders of the pancreas.

We wrote this book as a matter-of-fact reference for individuals and their families emphasizing the following important topics. We explain the role of the pancreas in the body's function, the various diseases that can affect the pancreas, how these conditions are diagnosed and treated, and how they affect your body's nutrition. We offer practical advice on how to live with the various disorders, including practical ways to prevent disease progression. Importantly, we try to simplify this often complex group of disorders so that patients can develop an appropriate understanding of their condition.

Living with pancreatic disease can be very challenging. While there have been significant advances in our understanding of why these diseases occur and breakthroughs in how they are treated, they still remain a mystery to many patients. It is our sincere hope that this book will help many take an important early step toward conquering their disease—the power of knowledge.

Timothy B. Gardner, MD
Andrew S. Warner, MD

PART ONE

The Basics

What is the digestive tract?

How is food digested?

What type of tests can be done to evaluate the digestive system?

More . . .

1. What is the digestive tract?

The digestive system (**Figure 1**) is a series of hollow organs joined in a long continuous tube—including the esophagus, stomach, and intestines—beginning in the mouth and ending in the **anus**. This tube is called the alimentary canal. Other abdominal organs—including the liver and pancreas—play a part in digestion. If it were to be uncoiled, the digestive tract would be about 30 feet long.

Anus

The outside opening of the rectum.

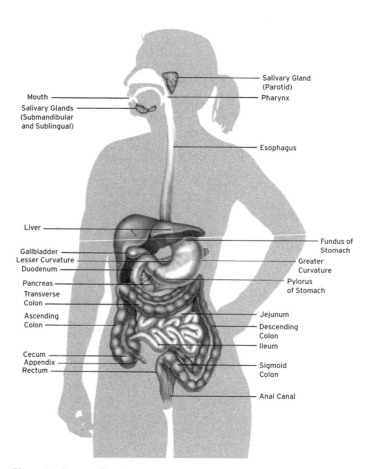

Figure 1 Human digestive system

The inside lining of these tubes is called **mucosa**. The mucosa contains glands, located in the mouth, stomach, and **small intestine**, which produce enzymes that aid in the digestion of food.

Though the liver, **gallbladder**, and pancreas are considered "solid organs" and not part of the alimentary canal, they are essential to digestive function.

The pancreas makes enzymes that work to digest proteins, fats, and carbohydrates. The pancreas also makes several chemicals, called hormones, which help with essential body functions. The most important of these chemicals is insulin. The liver produces **bile**, which is stored in the gallbladder. Bile is released from the gallbladder after eating to help absorb fat.

After food has been digested, the remaining waste travels from the small intestine to the **large intestine**. By the time food reaches the large intestine, all the essential nutrients have been absorbed by the small intestine. The large intestine works to remove water from the undigested material and form solid waste or stool.

The large intestine is made up of the **cecum**, ascending **colon**, transverse colon, descending colon, sigmoid colon, and **rectum**. The first part is the cecum, which is where the small intestine joins the large intestine. The last part is the rectum, where stool is stored until it leaves the digestive tract.

2. How is food digested?

Digestion is the process by which food is broken down in the **gastrointestinal tract**. Food that is useful to the

Mucosa
The innermost lining of the intestines.

Small intestine
The small bowel is made up of the duodenum, jejunum, and ileum.

Gallbladder
Pouch connected to the bile ducts that stores bile, which is released with eating to aid in digestion.

Bile
Thick, green fluid produced by the liver which plays an important role in the digestion of fats.

Large intestine
Also called colon; processes and stores waste.

Cecum
The first part of the large intestine; a pouch-like area into which the ileum opens.

Colon
The part of the large intestine that processes waste.

Rectum
Last part of colon where stool is stored until it leaves digestive tract.

Gastrointestinal tract
The digestive tube that starts at the mouth and ends at the anus.

The Basics

Absorption

The process of taking nutrients into the tissues.

body is brought into the body through a process called **absorption**. Food that is not needed for the body is eliminated in the form of stool and urine. In other words, digestion is the way that the body gets what it needs from food in order to stay healthy.

Digestion actually begins in the mouth with chewing. The purpose of chewing is to break food into smaller parts so that it can be swallowed. The **salivary glands** of the mouth release enzymes (chemicals which serve to break down food) in the form of saliva. Thus, the purpose of saliva is to assist in the breakdown of food while it is still in the mouth.

Salivary glands

Glands in the mouth that produce material that aid in the breakdown of food.

Oropharynx

Structure in the throat that connects directly with the beginning of the intestinal tract or esophagus.

Food travels from the mouth to the back of the throat (called the **oropharynx**) and then into the **esophagus**. The esophagus is a tube that connects the oropharynx to the stomach. Up until the food reaches the oropharynx, you can control the act of swallowing. However, once food reaches the esophagus, the digestive system's natural motor (the **motility system**) sweeps the food along the rest of the gastrointestinal tract.

Esophagus

Tube that carries food from the mouth to the stomach.

Motility system

The spontaneous contractions that move food through the gastrointestinal tract.

When the food reaches the stomach it is in a solid form. Once in the stomach, a very powerful chemical (stomach acid) breaks down the food into liquid form. Food can stay in the stomach anywhere from about an hour to about a day. Once the food is in a liquid form, it is then pushed into the small intestine where most of the absorption (taking vitamins and nutrients into the body so they can be used) occurs.

Duodenum

The first part of the small intestine, starting at the end of the stomach.

Jejunum

The middle section of the small intestine; between the duodenum and ileum.

The small intestine is a critical organ, as without it we would be unable to absorb the nutrition we need. The small intestine has three parts—the top part (**duodenum**), the middle part (the **jejunum**), and the end part (the **ileum**). Each part is lined with finger-like projections called **villi**. The villi are there to allow more nutrients to be absorbed into the body. At this point, the pancreas releases enzymes that work to break down and digest the food. As food travels down the small intestine, more and more nutrients are absorbed into the body.

Once the food has traveled through the small intestine, what is left over is solid waste and water, which then moves into the large intestine (or colon). It is the job of the colon to take in most of the water in the material so that by the time the food passes through the six-foot long colon and comes into the rectum, stool is formed. The rectum is the pouch which holds stool until there is a convenient time to have a bowel movement. Our conscious control over the digestion system returns when stool is in the rectum and one can sense the urge to have a bowel movement. The very end of the digestive system, the anus, is the opening of the rectum to the outside.

When food is swallowed and enters the gastrointestinal tract, it must travel between 25–30 feet before it reaches the anus. In other words, the intestinal tract in a typical adult is 25–30 feet long. As a result, in healthy patients, it typically takes at least 6–8 hours for food that is eaten to reach the end of the intestinal tract.

Sometimes, patients will notice that within a few minutes of eating they tend to have a bowel movement. Often patients will believe that "food goes right through me." While patients may have the sense that this is occurring, it is really impossible, given that the intestinal tract is so long. Much more likely is that the patient has a strong **gastrocolic reflex**. The gastrocolic

Ileum

Lowest section of the small intestine.

Villi

Finger-like projections lining the small intestine; involved in the digestion and absorption of food and nutrients.

The Basics

Gastrocolic reflex

A reflex in which the act of eating or food entering the stomach stimulates movement in the colon and/or small intestine.

5

Rapid intestinal transit

An increase in propulsion in the colon, such that the colon contracts more intensely than normal and food passes through more quickly.

Obstruction

A blockage of the small intestine or colon.

Perforation

A rupture or abnormal opening of the intestine that allows intestinal contents to escape into the abdominal cavity.

Abscess

A walled-off collection of pus; in Crohn's disease, an abscess is most commonly found around the anus or rectum, but can occur anywhere in the body.

Stricture

A narrowed area of intestine usually caused by scar tissue.

Fistula

A tunnel connecting two structures that are not normally connected.

Inflammation

A process characterized by swelling, warmth, redness, and/or tenderness; can occur in any organ.

reflex is a normal response to food going into the stomach. Food coming into the stomach can cause the colon to contract, which stimulates a bowel movement. This is not abnormal, although the reflex is stronger in some patients than in others.

Very rarely, patients will have food move through their intestinal tract faster than 6–8 hours. This process, called **rapid intestinal transit**, can occur in certain kinds of infections, swelling in the intestine, or cancers. However, rapid intestinal transit is rare and even still can take several hours for food taken in by mouth to reach the anus.

3. What type of tests can be done to evaluate the digestive system?

Healthcare providers may perform one or more tests to evaluate the digestive system. These include:

Abdominal X-ray: provides a picture of structures and organs in the abdomen and is helpful in detecting a bowel **obstruction** or a **perforation**.

CT scan: uses X-rays to create a more detailed look inside the body. It is especially helpful in detecting an **abscess**, and also useful in evaluating for a bowel obstruction or perforation.

Upper GI series/Upper GI series with small bowel follow through (SBFT): allows a close examination of the esophagus, stomach, duodenum, and small bowel by having the patient drink a thick, white liquid shake of barium, and then taking X-rays as it goes through the gastrointestinal tract. This is an excellent test to detect **strictures**, **fistulas**, and **inflammation** in the stomach and small bowel.

Barium enema: allows a close examination of the rectum and colon by instilling barium through the rectum and taking X-rays as it goes through the colon. This is an excellent test to detect strictures, inflammation, and fistulas in the colon.

Enteroclysis: provides a detailed examination of the small **bowel** by passing a small tube through the nose, into the stomach, and out into the duodenum. Barium is then instilled through the tube directly into the small bowel. This is an excellent test to detect abnormalities in the small intestine that may not have been seen on small bowel follow-through.

Ultrasound: uses sound waves to examine abdominal and pelvic organs. It is commonly used to look for **gallstones** and obstruction of the **bile duct**.

MRI: uses a magnetic field to create a detailed picture of the structures and organs in the abdomen and pelvis. This is especially helpful in detecting abdominal and pelvic abscesses; it can also be used to evaluate the bile duct and pancreatic duct.

Virtual colonoscopy: a CT scan of the colon used as a screening test for colon cancer as an alternative to endoscopy. This is increasingly being used, although it is unclear at present whether this is a better test than colonoscopy.

Upper endoscopy: usually performed under **sedation**; a small, thin, flexible, lighted tube with a camera on the end is passed through the mouth into the esophagus, stomach, and duodenum. This is an excellent test to detect inflammation and strictures in the upper GI tract, and allows for a **biopsy** to be taken.

Bowel

Another name for intestine.

Gallstones

Stones that form in the gallbladder.

Bile duct

A channel through which bile flows from the liver to the intestines.

Sedation

Also called conscious sedation, or moderate sedation; sedation is a form of moderate anesthesia in which the patient is given medication to induce a state of relaxation.

Biopsy

Usually performed during an endoscopy, a small piece of mucosa (inside lining of the intestine) is removed and examined under a microscope; an excellent test to characterize types of inflammation and detect dysplasia and cancer.

Colonoscopy: usually performed under sedation; a small, thin, flexible lighted tube with a camera on the end (called a colonoscope, see **Figure 2**) is passed through the rectum into the colon and, at times, the ileum. This is an excellent test to detect inflammation and strictures in the rectum, colon, and ileum, and allows for a biopsy to be taken.

Sigmoidoscopy: performed with or without sedation, this is a "short" colonoscopy used to examine the rectum and left colon.

Proctoscopy: performed without sedation, usually on a special tilt table that positions the patient with the head down and buttocks up. In this procedure a rigid, straight, lighted tube is used to examine the rectum. While this procedure has mostly been replaced by flexible sigmoidoscopy, this is still an excellent test to examine the rectum.

Anoscopy: performed without sedation, usually on a special tilt table that positions the patient with the head down and buttocks up. In this procedure a rigid, short, straight, lighted tube is used to examine the anal canal. This is an excellent test to examine for an anal fissure, or hemorrhoids.

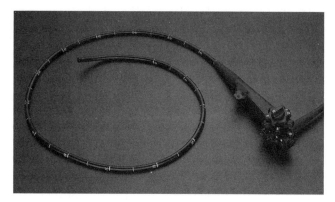

Figure 2   A colonoscope.

Enteroscopy: performed under sedation, a small, thin, long, flexible, lighted tube with a camera on the end is passed through the mouth into the esophagus, stomach, duodenum, and jejunum. This is an excellent test to detect inflammation and strictures in the upper GI tract and upper small intestine.

Capsule endoscopy: performed without sedation, the patient swallows a large pill containing a camera, and wears a sensor device on the abdomen. The capsule passes naturally through the small intestine while transmitting video images to the sensor which stores the data and can be downloaded to a computer for your physician to review. This test is mostly used in evaluating patients with **chronic** gastrointestinal bleeding of obscure origin. It is possible for the capsule, which is very large, to become lodged in an intestinal stricture and cause an obstruction; the patient would need an operation to remove the capsule.

Chronic

Usually refers to a disease that develops slowly and lasts for a long time.

Endoscopic retrograde cholangiopancreatography (ERCP): performed under sedation, this is an endoscopic procedure used to examine the bile duct and pancreatic duct. This procedure is performed for a variety of reasons including detection and removal of stones in the bile duct, detection of **tumors** involving the bile duct and pancreatic duct, and diagnosis of primary sclerosing **cholangitis**.

Tumor

An abnormal growth of tissue; can be benign or malignant.

Cholangitis

Infection of the bile ducts; can occur in primary sclerosing cholangitis (PSC).

Endoscopic ultrasound (EUS): performed under sedation, this is an endoscopic procedure used to examine the liver, bile ducts, esophagus, gallbladder, stomach, and pancreas. An EUS instrument is similar to one used for upper endoscopy, except that it is outfitted with an ultrasound machine in the end of the tube which allows for an "internal" ultrasound to

The Basics

be performed. The procedure is performed primarily to evaluate for tumors of these organs and can be a useful tool to obtain biopsies in hard-to-reach places in the abdomen or chest.

4. What is the pancreas and what does it do?

The pancreas is an oblong organ that sits in the upper abdomen. In the average adult it is typically between 6 and 10 inches long, 2 inches wide, and is located immediately behind the stomach and next to the duodenum (small intestine). It is divided into four parts: the head, body, tail, and **uncinate**.

Throughout the pancreas is a series of drainage tubes called the **pancreatic ducts**. The pancreas creates a "juice" comprised of digestive enzymes that are drained primarily by the main pancreatic duct, which empties into the duodenum at a site called the **ampulla of Vater**. This is also where bile draining from the liver and gallbladder empties into the duodenum. The tube that connects the liver and gallbladder to the duodenum is called the **common bile duct**. Thus, both the common bile duct (drains bile from the liver and gallbladder) and the main pancreatic duct (drains the pancreas) empty into the duodenum at the same location (**Figure 3**).

The functions of the pancreas can be divided into two main categories: **endocrine** and **exocrine**. The endocrine function involves specialized cells in the pancreas called **islet cells** that control the body's level of blood sugar. These cells produce hormones called **insulin** and **glucagon**, which are released directly into the bloodstream. The exocrine function involves cells in the

Uncinate

The part of the pancreas that wraps up under the "head" of the pancreas and sometimes circles the small intestine.

Pancreatic ducts

Drainage tubes of the pancreas.

Ampulla of Vater

Location of the major drainage from the pancreatic duct into the small intestine.

Common bile duct

Tube which connects the liver and gallbladder to the duodenum and drains bile into the small intestine.

Endocrine

Referring to the hormone-producing function of the pancreas.

Exocrine

Referring to the digestion function of the pancreas.

Islet cells

The microscopic parts of the pancreas which make hormones.

Insulin

A hormone made by the pancreas which helps to turn food into energy.

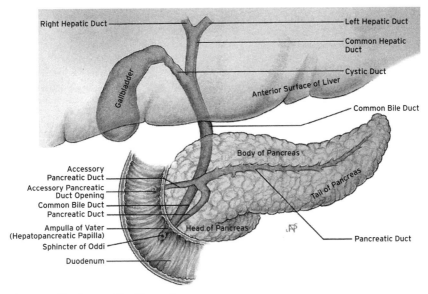

Figure 3   The liver, gallbadder, and pancreas.

pancreas which produce enzymes that aid in digestion of food. These enzymes are released into the main duct of the pancreas and then directly into the small intestine, where digestion takes place. Both functions of the pancreas are critical for health and wellness.

> **Glucagon**
>
> A hormone made by the pancreas which also helps to control blood sugar.

5. What are common diseases of the pancreas?

There is a variety of diseases that can lead to your pancreas not functioning properly. These are typically categorized into diseases that affect the exocrine (digestive) pancreas and the endocrine (hormonal) pancreas. Those diseases which affect the exocrine pancreas include pancreatitis (acute, chronic, hereditary, and autoimmune), pancreatic cancer, pancreatic cysts, cystic fibrosis, and pancreatic insufficiency. Those diseases which affect the endocrine pancreas include diabetes.

6. What are the symptoms of pancreatic diseases?

The symptoms of the different pancreatic diseases vary somewhat from disease to disease, although a common symptom among them is abdominal pain. The exceptions to this rule are diabetes and cystic fibrosis, which typically do not cause abdominal pain. Acute pancreatitis is notable for severe upper abdominal pain that radiates to the back, accompanied by nausea and vomiting, while those with chronic pancreatitis experience ongoing upper abdominal pain, weight loss, indigestion, and oily stools. **Table 1** lists several pancreatic diseases and their symptoms.

Table 1 Pancreatic Diseases Symptoms

Disease	Symptoms
Acute pancreatitis	Upper abdominal pain radiating to the back, nausea, vomiting, tender abdomen, may have fever
Chronic pancreatitis	Ongoing upper abdominal pain, weight loss, indigestion, oily stools
Hereditary pancreatitis	Similar in presentation to acute pancreatitis
Pancreatic cancer	Dark urine, pale bowel movements, itching, jaundice, weight loss, abdominal pain
Pancreatic cysts	Persistent abdominal pain, palpable mass, nausea, vomiting; however, may not experience any symptoms
Exocrine pancreatic insufficiency	Abdominal pain, weight loss, indigestion, oily stools
Diabetes	Frequent urination, excessive thirst, blurry vision, extreme fatigue, weight loss
Cystic fibrosis	Salty taste to skin, persistent cough, wheezing, weight loss (or poor weight gain in children), oily stools

7. What types of specialists do I see for pancreatic disease?

Your primary healthcare provider should be able to discern whether you should see a specialist and if so, what type of specialist you should see. You will likely be referred to a **gastroenterologist**—someone who specializes in disorders of the gastrointestinal tract (which includes the stomach, intestines, pancreas, liver, and gallbladder). Many of the tests used to diagnose pancreatic diseases are performed by a gastroenterologist.

Depending on your diagnosis, your primary healthcare provider might suggest you continue to see a gastroenterologist for treatment or might refer you to an endocrinologist, a doctor that specializes in disorders relating to the glands and hormones. If you are diagnosed with pancreatic cancer, you will likely see an **oncologist**—a clinician who specializes in cancer detection and treatment.

Gastro-enterologist

A physician who specializes in diseases of the gastro-intestinal tract, liver, and pancreas.

Oncologist

A physician whose area of expertise is diagnosis and treatment of tumors.

The Basics

PART TWO

The Pancreas and Gallbladder

What is acute pancreatitis?

How is acute pancreatitis diagnosed?

What causes acute pancreatitis?

More . . .

8. What is acute pancreatitis?

The major type of chemical made by the pancreas for digestion is pancreatic enzymes. These enzymes are used by the body to break down fats, carbohydrates, and proteins within the small intestine so that they can be absorbed into the bloodstream. The pancreatic enzymes primarily responsible for digesting fats are called **lipases**, and the pancreatic enzymes primarily responsible for digesting proteins are called **proteases**. The pancreatic enzymes primarily responsible for digesting starches are called **amylases**.

Lipases

Pancreatic enzymes that digest fats.

Proteases

Pancreatic enzymes that digest proteins.

Amylases

Pancreatic enzymes that digest starches.

The pancreatic enzymes produced in the pancreas are very powerful; so much so that they are wrapped in a protective covering when they are within the pancreas. When food is eaten and travels to the stomach, a signal is sent to release the pancreas enzymes into the small intestine through the pancreas ductal system. It is only when the enzymes reach the small intestine and are completely out of the pancreas that the covering is removed by a chemical in the small intestine, called **enterokinase**. In this manner, the enzymes are only activated and able to digest food when they are outside of the pancreas. When pancreas enzymes become prematurely unwrapped (activated) while they are still inside the pancreas, they begin to digest the pancreas. This process of **autodigestion** of the pancreas by pancreatic enzymes is what causes acute pancreatitis.

Enterokinase

A chemical within the small intestine which allows the pancreas enzymes to be unwrapped and begin digesting food.

Autodigestion

The process by which prematurely activated pancreatic enzymes digest the pancreas, leading to acute pancreatitis.

When acute pancreatitis occurs, the pancreas becomes inflamed and patients generally develop severe abdominal pain fairly suddenly. The pain is most often located in the center of the upper abdomen, between the navel and the lower end of the breastbone, but can also occur in the upper abdomen on the left or right side. The pain can also occur lower in the abdomen, at about the level of the navel.

The pain often bores through from the front of the abdomen to the back. In many cases, the pain is accompanied by nausea and vomiting and patients may develop a fever. Patients generally see a healthcare provider within a day or so of the onset of the pain. Often, the severity of the pain prompts a visit to the emergency room.

Most cases of acute pancreatitis require admission to the hospital. However, the majority of the time, even though the initial symptoms are quite severe, the situation improves quickly and patients stay in the hospital for only a few days. Less commonly, the pain persists, requiring a longer stay in the hospital.

About one in ten cases of acute pancreatitis is more serious. The inflammation of the pancreas will lead to impairment in lung or kidney function or infection. These issues may in turn require transfer to an intensive care unit. Sometimes a breathing tube or kidney dialysis is needed. Severe cases of acute pancreatitis can be life-threatening.

Severe acute pancreatitis may lead to death of pancreatic tissue. This dead tissue can become infected, which is potentially fatal. This type of infection may not be treatable with antibiotics alone, but instead requires surgery to remove the infected tissue. Large collections of fluid called **pseudocysts** can also develop when pancreatitis is severe.

Pseudocyst
Fluid-filled collection of tissue in or adjacent to the pancreas.

9. How is acute pancreatitis diagnosed?

Acute pancreatitis is suspected by the healthcare provider when a patient describes the sudden development of severe pain in the upper abdomen. Because pancreatitis is usually caused by either alcohol intake or gallstones, the suspicion for acute pancreatitis is increased when the patient has ingested alcohol, or when the patient is known to have gallstones.

The physical examination is important in diagnosing acute pancreatitis. Patients generally appear uncomfortable from the pain and nausea. There may be a rapid heart rate or elevated blood pressure from the pain, nausea and vomiting, and dehydration. There may also be a mild fever. Examination of the upper abdomen reveals tenderness, which may be severe.

Because the pancreas releases its enzymes into the bloodstream during acute pancreatitis, detection of elevation in these enzymes is crucial for the diagnosis of acute pancreatitis. The most common blood tests are the amylase and lipase level. These are enzymes produced by the pancreas that spill into the bloodstream during acute pancreatitis. It is normal to have some amylase or lipase in the bloodstream; however, the levels of at least one of these enzymes should be at least three times the maximum normal level in order to clinch the diagnosis of acute pancreatitis. The amylase and lipase tests each have advantages and disadvantages. The amylase is elevated earlier in the illness, which is more useful since most patients come to their healthcare provider soon after the pain begins. However, elevation in amylase is not unique to acute pancreatitis (i.e., amylase may be elevated in other gastrointestinal disorders such as gallbladder infection). Furthermore, amylase is also normally found in saliva, and disorders of the salivary glands can also raise the level of amylase in the blood and confuse the issue. Lipase is more specific to the pancreas, but the level of lipase may rise later in the illness and thus is not always as helpful in the early setting.

Radiologic imaging of the abdomen is also very important in diagnosing acute pancreatitis. What particular test is ordered by the healthcare provider may depend on the hospital. An ultrasound, CT scan, and MRI are all capable of diagnosing acute pancreatitis. These tests can each identify the hallmarks of acute pancreatitis, which are swelling or enlargement of the pancreas and abnormal fluid around the pancreas. Each test has advantages and disadvantages—you can discuss these with your healthcare provider.

10. What causes acute pancreatitis?

More than 80% of cases of acute pancreatitis in the United States are caused by either alcohol or gallstones. Alcohol has a damaging effect on the pancreas and can trigger the process of autodigestion. The amount of ingested alcohol necessary to cause acute pancreatitis is generally large. Most patients who have acute pancreatitis related to alcohol drink considerable amounts of alcohol on a chronic basis (e.g., 6 drinks a day for 10–15 years); however, lesser amounts can cause pancreatitis as well. The attack of acute pancreatitis typically occurs within a few days of alcohol ingestion.

Gallstones or thick bile (called sludge) are frequent causes of acute pancreatitis. This occurs when a gallstone or thick sludge escapes from the gallbladder into the bile duct. The bile duct joins with the duct from the pancreas just before both ducts empty into the small intestine. When a gallstone or sludge blocks the pancreatic duct, pancreatitis can result. Because the bile duct and the pancreatic duct are small, it is usually small gallstones that cause acute pancreatitis.

In addition to alcohol and gallstone disease, there are several other, less common reasons patients can develop acute pancreatitis (see **Table 2** for both common and rare causes). Any condition which causes a blockage of the pancreatic duct, such as a mass due to pancreatic cancer or a **pancreatic cyst** (a fluid-filled sac in the pancreas), can cause pancreatitis. Fortunately, the vast majority of patients with acute pancreatitis do not have pancreatic cancer. In some patients, an elevation in the blood stream of **triglycerides** can cause acute pancreatitis. Triglycerides are a type of fat, related to cholesterol, which makes the blood oftentimes very thick. When the triglyceride count is high, the blood has trouble carrying enough oxygen to the pancreas, and this can lead to acute pancreatitis. Many medications can cause pancreatitis, and usually the pancreatitis starts after being on the medication for only a short time. Pancreatitis may also result from a type of endoscopy looking at the pancreas called an ERCP. This procedure involves injecting a special contrast dye into the pancreas and/or bile ducts and is often performed to evaluate for possible stones in the bile or pancreas ducts. This procedure typically causes acute pancreatitis in about 5% of the patients undergoing the test. High calcium levels, viral infections, celiac disease, and trauma can also cause acute pancreatitis.

Pancreatic cyst

A fluid-filled cavity in the pancreas that can sometimes cause acute pancreatitis if it is blocking the pancreatic duct.

Triglycerides

A type of fat found in the bloodstream.

11. How is acute pancreatitis treated?

Patients are usually admitted to the hospital for treatment of acute pancreatitis. Treatment of acute pancreatitis is supportive. A principle of treatment is resting the pancreas; because the pancreas is stimulated by eating, patients are treated with "nothing by mouth" (or NPO) initially. In order to maintain adequate

Table 2   Causes of Acute Pancreatitis

Common Causes	Comments
Excessive alcohol use	Accounts for about 40% of all causes of acute pancreatitis. Usually >6 drinks per day for 10–15 years, although can be from less use. Occasionally can occur after first time use
Gallbladder stones or sludge	Accounts for about 40% of all causes of acute pancreatitis. Usually small gallstones that cause pancreatitis
Occasional Causes	
High triglycerides	A type of fat in the blood; high levels which cause pancreatitis are usually due in part to having hereditary high triglyceride levels
Medications	Many medications can cause acute pancreatitis, including estrogens, certain antibiotics, and some medications to treat AIDS
Pancreatic cysts or cancer	These conditions cause blockages of the tube (pancreatic duct) which drains the pancreas
Post-ERCP	Acute pancreatitis occurs in about 5% of patients who undergo an ERCP test
Rare Causes	
High blood calcium levels	This occurs usually when someone has another type of cancer such as breast cancer, or in patients with over-functioning parathyroid glands
Celiac disease	Can occur in patients with celiac disease—an allergy to the gluten component of wheat, barley and rye
Hereditary pancreatitis	The tendency to develop acute pancreatitis can be passed down from family members
Autoimmune pancreatitis	The body's own immune system can attack the pancreas, causing acute pancreatitis

hydration, intravenous fluids are given. Dehydration may be compounded by loss of fluids from vomiting. The pain from acute pancreatitis can be intense, and so narcotics are given intravenously. Medication for nausea is also given. If vomiting is persistent, a plastic tube may be placed from the nose to the stomach to remove fluid from the stomach (a **nasogastric** or "NG tube"), although this does not specifically target the inflammation of the pancreas. However, with the supportive treatment outlined above, patients usually get better in a few days and are discharged from the hospital.

Nasogastric tube

A long, flexible tube that is passed through the nose into the stomach and is used to suction out the stomach in the setting of a bowel obstruction or sometimes after an operation.

The Pancreas and Gallbladder

21

In a minority of cases, acute pancreatitis can become severe. Blood pressure can become dangerously low. There can be impairment of lung and kidney function and a serious infection may develop. In these cases, careful monitoring in the intensive care unit is mandatory. If the impairment in lung function is severe enough, placement of a breathing tube may be necessary. In some cases, dialysis is needed due to kidney failure. In severe cases of acute pancreatitis, some or all of the pancreatic tissue dies. This dead pancreatic tissue is at high risk for becoming infected. When infection of this tissue occurs, treatment with antibiotics alone is not sufficient and surgery is necessary. Fluid-filled collections of tissue called pseudocysts may form. These can also become infected, or they can block the flow of nutrients through the digestive tract. These pseudocysts can be treated with surgery or with a special type of drainage procedure performed either with an endoscopy whereby the pseudocyst is drained through the stomach, or a specialized radiologist will place a drain in the pseudocyst under CT scan guidance.

There is a role for a specialized type of endoscopy called an ERCP in some cases of acute pancreatitis related to gallstones. When the gastroenterologist believes that the gallstone is stuck in the bile duct where it joins the pancreatic duct, he or she may recommend an ERCP to prevent an infection from forming in the bile duct. Performing this specialized procedure, the gastroenterologist advances a flexible endoscope into the small intestine at the point where the bile duct and pancreatic duct join and drain into the small intestine. A catheter is threaded into the opening of these ducts and the opening is enlarged using a technique called **sphincterotomy**. The stone is pulled out and allowed to pass through the intestine.

Sphincterotomy

A surgical procedure to open a muscle sphincter wide enough for gallstones to pass through.

12. How do I prevent acute pancreatitis?

The most important way to prevent acute pancreatitis is to try to determine, with the help of your gastroenterologist, the underlying cause of the problem. For example, if excessive alcohol use is the cause, it is imperative that you completely avoid alcohol use in the future. It is essential to view alcohol almost as an allergy—that your body cannot tolerate alcohol because you are allergic to it. If gallbladder disease is the cause, then having your gallbladder removed (called a **cholecystectomy**) may be the most appropriate treatment option. Please talk with your doctor about the right treatment for you. It is important to stop taking medications if they are believed to be the cause of the pancreatitis. However, do not stop taking any medications without consulting with your healthcare provider. High triglycerides, if found to be the cause of pancreatitis, can generally be treated with medications.

Preventing pancreatitis related to an ERCP procedure is often difficult. Typically, no matter the experience level of the gastroenterologist performing the ERCP, the rate of pancreatitis resulting from this procedure is around 3–5%. It is important for you and your clinician to make sure that the ERCP is being performed for a good reason and that you are aware, before undergoing the procedure, that there is a risk of pancreatitis.

In addition, the following general principles apply. Try to maintain a healthy lifestyle with frequent weekly exercise and a diet which has at least 5 servings of fruits and vegetables daily. If you are a smoker, try and quit, as it is becoming increasingly clear that smoking may play a role in making the pancreas more likely to

Cholecystectomy
Surgical removal of the gallbladder.

become inflamed. This also includes avoiding second-hand smoke. Trying to stay hydrated with at least 8 glasses of water daily is also important.

Despite these measures, if you develop an attack, it is essential to seek medical attention quickly, especially if you cannot take in any fluids. This is important because the more dehydrated you become, the more likely you are to have a severe bout of pancreatitis. Coming to the emergency room or your healthcare provider's office early after developing symptoms can be key to helping prevent severe pancreas damage and a prolonged hospitalization.

Patient Perspective

Sally is a 45-year-old mother of three who works as a kindergarten teacher. For the past several weeks, she has been feeling occasional sharp pain in the right upper part of her abdomen about 30 minutes after eating. The pain lasts for a few hours and then goes away slowly. She notices that the pain seems to be the worst after she eats fatty meals like pizza. She kept meaning to see her doctor, but between work and the kids, she kept putting off the appointment.

Earlier this evening, after Sunday dinner at her mother's house, she developed a new kind of pain. The pain was located in the center of her abdomen and moved toward her back. She could not find a comfortable position and over the course of the next several hours the pain got worse and worse until she went to the emergency room. The pain felt more intense than her previous pain attacks and was not going away. In the emergency room she was given pain medication and had blood tests taken. The doctor in the emergency room told Sally that she had pancreatitis after reviewing her blood tests and admitted her to the hospital.

She was not allowed to eat and she was given a lot of fluid through her intravenous (IV) line in her arm. She was also given medications to help treat her pain. After three days her pain started to go away and her appetite returned. She had an ultrasound test performed of her gallbladder which revealed small stones. She was seen by a surgeon who told Sally that her pancreatitis was due to a gallstone. On the fourth day of her hospitalization, she had her gallbladder removed to prevent any further attacks of pancreatitis. She did very well and was discharged home the next day. She has not had any further attacks of pain since the surgery.

Healthcare Provider Perspective

Sally had classic symptoms of biliary colic, in which the gallbladder and bile ducts were put under pressure after she ate a fatty meal. This pain is usually located in the right upper part of the abdomen where these organs are located and is due to the squeezing of the gallbladder and bile ducts against a blockage; in this case a stone. Sally's pain would improve after a few hours because the stone would pass into the small intestine or become dislodged from the ampulla.

She developed pancreatitis because the stone got lodged in the opening of the ampulla of Vater, where both the pancreas and bile ducts drain into the small intestine. The stone had travelled out of the gallbladder into the bile duct. When the stone became lodged at the ampulla of Vater, it caused back pressure in her pancreas, leading to pancreatitis. The reason why the character of her

> *pain changed was because when she came into the hospital, she had developed pancreatitis.*
>
> *Her acute pancreatitis was treated appropriately with pain medication, lots of intravenous fluids, and avoiding eating. About 80% of the time patients develop acute pancreatitis, the pancreatitis will calm down without causing any long-term damage. However, 15–20% of the time the pancreatitis can cause damage to other organs, and 5% of the time pancreatitis can be fatal.*
>
> *The treatment of Sally's acute pancreatitis was removing the gallbladder because it was the stone in the gallbladder which caused the pancreatitis. It was correct to have the surgery before she left the hospital because many patients who are sent home before their gallbladder is removed have to return due to repeat bouts of pancreatitis. Sally should not have any further attacks of pancreatitis in the future now that the gallbladder has been removed.*

13. What is chronic pancreatitis?

Chronic pancreatitis is a chronic inflammatory condition which results in destruction of the pancreatic tissue. Depending on the severity of the case, varying amounts of the pancreas are destroyed. This condition is often very painful, debilitating, and difficult to treat.

Some recent research indicates that about half of chronic pancreatitis cases are due to alcohol consumption. In most of these cases, patients with chronic pancreatitis from alcohol have consumed large amounts of alcohol for many years. Other causes of chronic pancreatitis include cigarette smoking, obstruction, genetic factors, and idiopathic pancreatitis (arising from an unknown cause). Rarer causes include hyper-triglyceridemia and tropical pancreatitis (which is found only in a few specific locations, such as India). There is a rare, hereditary form of chronic pancreatitis. The genes responsible for this disorder have been iden-tified. In contrast to chronic pancreatitis, which gener-ally afflicts individuals in early adulthood and middle age, hereditary pancreatitis strikes earlier in life. Much attention has also been given to cystic fibrosis as a cause of chronic pancreatitis. Individuals who do not have the full-blown disease of cystic fibrosis, but carry one of the two genes necessary for the disease (called **heterozygotes**), may have chronic pancreatitis but no other signs of cystic fibrosis.

Heterozygote

An individual who has two different forms of a particular gene (one normal, the other either dominant or recessive).

The type of damage to the pancreas that occurs in chronic pancreatitis is variable and unpredictable. Sometimes the inflammation is on a microscopic level and difficult to see with radiologic tests such as CT scans. In other cases, the pancreas is obviously inflamed and destroyed. The main pancreatic duct is often abnormally enlarged or alternatively may have narrowed areas called strictures. There may be cal-cium deposits in the pancreas tissue which can be seen even with a standard X-ray of the abdomen. Some-times plugs of thick material can accumulate in the pancreatic duct and block the outflow of pancreatic enzymes, thereby contributing to the pain. In up to half of patients with chronic pancreatitis, the pancreas becomes damaged to the point that it is no longer able to produce the pancreas enzymes necessary to digest food (and therefore, fat) properly. When this hap-pens the patient is not getting the proper vitamins and nutrients from the food they eat, leading to malnutri-tion and malabsorption, and in some cases, unintended weight loss.

14. How is chronic pancreatitis diagnosed?

Healthcare providers suspect chronic pancreatitis in patients with severe pain in the upper abdomen, particularly those with a history of excessive alcohol intake. However, not all patients with chronic pancreatitis have a history of alcohol abuse. As in acute pancreatitis, the pain of chronic pancreatitis will often radiate to the back and can be triggered by eating. Other signs and symptoms to suggest chronic pancreatitis include unintentional weight loss and evidence of oily, foul-smelling stools (called **steatorrhea**), which result from loss of pancreatic digestive enzymes.

Steatorrhea

The presence of excess fat in the stool.

Unlike acute pancreatitis, in which the amylase and/or lipase are elevated, in chronic pancreatitis the amylase and lipase blood levels are usually normal. In severe chronic pancreatitis, impairment of digestion is confirmed by collection of stool for 3 days and measuring the fat content. Obviously, this test is inconvenient to perform and the results may be normal in mild or moderate cases. Tests to check pancreas enzyme levels in the stool are also limited in that they tend to be elevated only in severe cases of chronic pancreatitis, when the diagnosis was never in doubt in the first place.

The diagnosis of chronic pancreatitis is generally confirmed by some type of imaging test to visualize the pancreas. A routine X-ray of the abdomen may demonstrate calcium deposits in the pancreas, a sign of chronic pancreatitis. More commonly, a CT scan or an MRI is necessary to confirm the diagnosis. The findings of chronic pancreatitis are variable. These imaging tests may show inflammation or atrophy of the pancreas. The main duct draining the pancreatic juice (called the pancreatic duct) may be widened, or may show concentrated areas of narrowing or stones within the duct. An MRI is particularly useful for evaluating the pancreatic duct.

An ERCP can also be used as a diagnostic test to identify the abnormalities of the pancreatic duct seen in chronic pancreatitis. However, an MRI provides nearly the same information without the risk of an invasive procedure, so it has largely replaced an ERCP as the best diagnostic test for evaluating the pancreatic duct.

Increasingly, an endoscopic ultrasound (EUS) is being used as the gold standard test to diagnose chronic pancreatitis because it is a simple test that is very sensitive for detecting changes in the pancreas. The limitation of an EUS is that it is not widely available and its accuracy depends on the skill of the physician performing the test.

15. How is chronic pancreatitis treated?

The treatment of chronic pancreatitis is challenging. The goals of treatment are reduction of pain and treatment of weight loss and malnutrition. The pain from chronic pancreatitis is usually severe enough to require strong pain-killing medication, frequently narcotics. Initially, over-the-counter analgesics are tried but are generally ineffective. In severe cases, strong narcotics are necessary to control the pain. In patients with intermittent pain, the healthcare provider prescribes medication to take on an as-needed basis only when the pain occurs. In patients with chronic pain, the provider prescribes long-acting narcotics to take on a daily basis, in the hope of making the pain manageable or preventing pain before it starts.

Pancreatic enzymes are prescribed and are effective in treating the impaired digestion that occurs in severe chronic pancreatitis, and in this way are able to target the weight loss, malnutrition, and malabsorption experienced by many patients. The replacement enzymes aid in absorbing the vitamins and nutrients from food the patient eats. Often, a medication to suppress acid production from the stomach is prescribed in conjunction with the enzymes, in order to prevent stomach acid from breaking down the enzymes in the stomach.

In selected cases there is a role for endoscopic or surgical treatment of chronic pancreatitis. In some cases of chronic pancreatitis, stones form in the pancreatic duct and can block the flow of pancreatic juice into the small intestine. This blockage can contribute to the pain in this condition. An ERCP can be used to remove the stones from the main pancreatic duct. Sometimes a technique called **extracorporeal shock-wave lithotripsy (ESWL)** is used first to fragment the stones into smaller pieces so that they can be more easily removed by an ERCP. This technique is often performed by urologists because it is most commonly used in the treatment of kidney stones.

Extracorporeal shock wave lithotripsy (ESWL)

Noninvasive technique using high-energy sound waves to break up gallstones.

If initial measures are unsuccessful and symptoms are disabling, surgery may be considered for chronic pancreatitis. Surgery is not a suitable option for chronic pancreatitis in all cases. There are different operations that the surgeon will consider. Surgery on the pancreas can be complex and carry significant risk. It is recommended that patients choose a surgeon who specializes in diseases of the pancreas and has experience in pancreatic surgery.

16. How do I prevent chronic pancreatitis?

The single most important way to prevent chronic pancreatitis is to avoid the trigger of the disease, if possible. For many patients, this means completely stopping the use of all alcohol and tobacco products as both have been shown to be major triggers of chronic pancreatitis. It is not felt to be beneficial to just limit the amount of alcohol and tobacco use—completely stopping is the only way to avoid the harms of these triggers.

In addition, many people develop chronic pancreatitis from having repeated attacks of acute pancreatitis. Because of this, it is very important to identify the cause of the acute pancreatitis and treat it so that further attacks don't occur. For example, if you have high triglyceride levels in the blood which causes acute pancreatitis, these levels should be lowered with medications to avoid any further attacks.

Many patients who have chronic pancreatitis will develop **exocrine pancreatic insufficiency (EPI)**. It is critical for these patients to avoid diets high in fat, as this can worsen symptoms. However, if you have been prescribed pancreas enzyme replacement therapy (PERT), take them regularly with meals to prevent nutritional complications. Taking PERT, as prescribed by your physician, will allow you to get back to a normal diet and return to what your regular fat intake was. PERT should also be taken with food since this therapy is intended to do the digestive work that normal pancreas enzymes do with food intake.

Exocrine pancreatic insufficiency (EPI)

When the pancreas fails to produce enough digestive enzymes to support adequate nutrient absorption.

For some patients, however, the trigger for chronic pancreatitis cannot be identified. In these situations, it is critical to maintain a healthy lifestyle, including limiting fatty food intake, eating a diet rich in fruits and vegetables, and generally limiting alcohol and tobacco use.

Patient Perspective

Jim is a 52-year-old accountant who three months ago began to notice an ache in the center of his abdomen above his belly button. The pain initially would come on 1–2 times per week and last for a few hours. He could not identify any obvious trigger to the pain, such as what he ate or what he was doing when the pain started. In the last month, however, the pain has become more chronic. It is so severe that he has had to miss a few days of work. The pain also seems to have traveled to his mid back as well as in his abdomen. He has noticed that his appetite is no longer as good as it once was, and he thinks he has lost about 5 pounds in the last month.

Jim does have a strong family history of pancreas disease. His father died from pancreatic cancer, and his uncle has chronic pancreatitis. Jim does not drink alcohol, but does smoke a pack of cigarettes per day.

Jim went to his doctor, and after hearing Jim's story the doctor became concerned about the diagnosis of chronic pancreatitis and ordered a CT scan. The CT scan showed that Jim's pancreas had many small stones in it and was also smaller than would be expected in someone his age. Jim had many questions for his doctor about how he got chronic pancreatitis and what he could do to help relieve the pain.

Healthcare Provider Perspective

Jim has a fairly typical story for a patient with chronic pancreatitis. Many cases of chronic pancreatitis can be caused by familial or genetic causes. In fact, most cases of chronic pancreatitis are probably in some way influenced by traits that were passed down by a patient's parents. Both alcohol consumption and smoking also appear to be closely related to the development of chronic pancreatitis. For some patients, the amount of alcohol can be as little as 3–4 drinks per day for 10 years; for other patients, the amount can be considerably more. However, it is important to recognize that every patient is different, and that doctors are not entirely sure of why it takes differing amounts of alcohol consumption or tobacco use in patients to cause chronic pancreatitis.

In addition to genetic causes, alcohol consumption and tobacco use, recurrent bouts of acute pancreatitis, hereditary pancreatitis (that which is passed on between family members), or blockages of the drainage tubes of the pancreas can also cause chronic pancreatitis. It is essential that Jim's healthcare provider make sure that he does not have any of these other conditions that could be contributing to his disease.

The best treatment for Jim at this time is to completely stop using tobacco products. Many patients with chronic pancreatitis get relief from their symptoms by simply stopping the toxins which are hurting the pancreas.

If medications do not work to help control the pain, stronger pain medications are often required. Opiates, or narcotics, are strong pain relievers that can be used to treat the pain from chronic pancreatitis. However, they have two major side effects. The first is that they are generally very addictive and thus it is important to have these medications managed closely by a health-care provider. The second is that patients often develop tolerance to the medications—that is, it takes more and more of the medications over time to maintain the same level of pain control.

Overall, it will be very important for Jim to make a real change in his life in regard to his tobacco use, in addition to maintaining a close relationship with his healthcare provider to maximize his treatment for this disease.

17. What is autoimmune pancreatitis?

Autoimmune pancreatitis is a type of chronic pancreatitis which has recently been identified. The term autoimmune refers to the fact that the damage to the pancreas is caused by the body's own immune system, the system which helps the body fight infections. Rather than strictly fighting infections targeted against the body, for unknown reasons the immune system actually attacks the pancreas.

Jaundice

Yellowing of the skin due to buildup of bile.

Most patients with autoimmune pancreatitis come to medical attention because their skin turns yellow (**jaundice**) due to blockage of that part of the bile duct which travels through the pancreas. Often, there is a mass present within the pancreas, leading healthcare providers to be concerned about the development of pancreatic cancer. Patients can also come to medical attention because they develop repeated attacks of acute pancreatitis or develop pancreatic exocrine insufficiency.

Autoimmune pancreatitis is usually diagnosed based on findings on a CT scan and a specialized blood test called an IgG4 level. Since autoimmune pancreatitis can be associated with other autoimmune conditions such as **colitis** (inflammation of the colon) or **Sjögren's syndrome** (drying of the glands that make saliva), it is sometimes found in the process of evaluating these other diseases.

Autoimmune pancreatitis is unique because it is the one type of chronic pancreatitis that can be effectively reversed with medication. The treatment of autoimmune pancreatitis is with short courses of medications called **corticosteroids**.

It is important to remember, however, that autoimmune pancreatitis is a very rare disease. Unfortunately, it is much more likely for a patient to have pancreatic cancer or "typical" chronic pancreatitis than autoimmune pancreatitis. Nevertheless, autoimmune pancreatitis should always be considered as a possible diagnosis in a patient who has other autoimmune diseases and in whom, after extensive evaluation, a diagnosis of cancer cannot be made.

18. What is hereditary pancreatitis?

Hereditary pancreatitis is a rare, inherited condition that affects the exocrine function of the pancreas. Scientists have found that individuals with this disorder have a mutation (change) in the cationic trypsinogen gene (PRSS1), the gene responsible for producing the enzyme that breaks down proteins in the food we eat.

Colitis

Inflammation of the colon; can be due to Crohn's disease, ulcerative colitis, or other diseases.

Sjögren's syndrome

A disorder of the immune system that affects the body's production of tears and saliva.

Corticosteroids

A type of medication given to reduce inflammation. Corticosteroids come in oral and topical forms.

The Pancreas and Gallbladder

Similar to chronic pancreatitis, hereditary pancreatitis is marked by repeated episodes of acute pancreatitis, which eventually leads to a diagnosis of chronic pancreatitis. In patients whose pancreatitis attacks started before age 20 or who have family histories of close relatives with chronic pancreatitis, genetic testing can confirm the diagnosis.

Treatment of hereditary pancreatitis is the same as that for chronic pancreatitis, with pain control and a prescription of pancreas enzymes being the primary interventions. Unfortunately, hereditary pancreatitis greatly increases the lifetime risk of developing pancreatic cancer.

19. What is the gallbladder?

The gallbladder is a green, pear-shaped organ that sits next to the liver in the right upper abdomen. It is about 3 to 5 inches long. The function of the gallbladder is to store bile produced by the liver. The gallbladder contracts and releases bile into the intestine after meals. Bile has an important role in digesting fats. Despite these important-sounding functions, humans can live normal, healthy lives if the gallbladder has to be removed surgically (most often due to gallstones, which are addressed in Question 20). The functions of the gallbladder are assumed by the liver and bile ducts after the gallbladder has been removed.

20. What are gallstones and how are they treated?

Gallstones range in size from tiny particles like grains of sand up to firm concretions 2 inches in diameter.

Sometimes a jelly-like material forms which is called gallbladder sludge. Although sludge is liquid and stones are solid, sludge can cause the very same problems as stones. Most gallstones are cholesterol stones, which are composed primarily of cholesterol. A minority of stones are pigment stones, which are made up of multiple components of bile, including calcium and **bilirubin**. These substances naturally occur in bile.

Gallstones form when there is an imbalance in the components of bile. This results in solid material precipitating out of the bile to form stones.

Bilirubin
Product of the breakdown of hemoglobin, which can be measured to evaluate the liver and gallbladder.

Who is at risk for developing stones? The risk factors for cholesterol and pigment stones are different. Women are two to three times as likely as men to develop cholesterol stones. Pregnancy is a risk factor for gallstones. Certain ethnic groups such as Native Americans have a higher rate of gallstones. African-Americans are less likely than whites to develop gallstones. Both obesity and rapid weight loss have been associated with gallstone formation. Because gallstones rarely disappear on their own, they are more commonly seen in older people. Several drugs, most notably female hormones, increase the risk of gallstone formation.

The risk factors for pigment stones are different from cholesterol stones. Pigment stones account for no more than 25% of stones in the United States, but they account for a much higher percentage of gallstones among Asian-Americans. Risk factors for pigment stones include blood disorders in which red blood cells are destroyed, releasing bilirubin, which creates an imbalance in the composition of bile leading to stone precipitation. **Cirrhosis** of the liver can also lead to pigment stones. Some individuals have chronic

Cirrhosis
Formation of permanent scar tissue in the liver due to a chronic condition.

infection of the bile ducts, which is known to cause pigment stones. This condition is much more common in Asia than the United States.

Although the cholesterol and pigment stones are different in terms of how they are formed, once formed they cause very similar problems.

The best treatment for gallstones in the gallbladder is surgery. Once the gallbladder is removed, most patients have no further problems from gallstones. The risk of problems following gallbladder removal does not decline to zero, however, because stones can form in the bile duct. Unlike the gallbladder, the bile duct is essential for survival and cannot be removed.

The traditional operation for removing the gallbladder involves making an incision in the right upper abdomen. This operation is tried and true but requires several days in the hospital and about one month before returning to work.

This surgery, often called "open" cholecystectomy (removal of the gallbladder), has been replaced by laparoscopic cholecystectomy as the "gold standard" for the treatment of gallstones. In this operation, the surgeon removes the gallbladder without a large incision. Instead, four much smaller incisions are made and the gallbladder is removed with the use of a video camera and other specialized instruments. The laparoscopic approach is still surgery and requires general anesthesia. However, because of the much smaller incisions, patients usually can either go home the same day of the operation or sometimes stay one night in the hospital. Patients typically return to work in one to two weeks.

The obvious advantages of the laparoscopic approach to removing the gallbladder make this the first choice for both patients and physicians. But in some cases the laparoscopic approach is not possible and the surgeon has no choice but to open the abdomen and perform the traditional operation. For example, a large amount of scar tissue in the abdomen can obstruct the surgeon's ability to dissect the gallbladder out safely using the laparoscopic technique.

Surgery is the preferred option for the vast majority of patients with problems related to gallstones. A problem arises when a patient is felt to be too high a risk to undergo an operation or if the patient is opposed to having surgery. There are a few other options available. In a patient with an infected gallbladder (**acute cholecystitis**), who is believed to be at high risk for surgery, the radiologist may insert a tube through the skin into the gallbladder, called a percutaneous **cholecystostomy**. This tube will drain the infection and together with antibiotics can provide temporary treatment.

Acute cholecystitis

An inflammation of the gallbladder, most often due to gallstones, marked by severe abdominal pain and may be accompanied by fever.

Cholecystostomy

Drainage tube placed through the skin directly into the gallbladder.

Another option is medical therapy in the form of pills to dissolve stones. This treatment was more popular before the advent of laparoscopic surgery. The prescribed medication changes the composition of bile and can dissolve gallstones. Unfortunately, only a fraction of patients with gallstones are even candidates for this form of treatment. Patients must take medication for up to 2 years and even then the medication is successful only about half the time. And over several years after stopping treatment, stones will re-form in 50% of individuals.

Extracorporeal shock-wave lithotripsy (ESWL) has been used as an alternative to surgery, with medical therapy prescribed afterward. This treatment, like medical therapy alone, is limited by the high rate of recurrent problems after the treatment is discontinued. Surgery is the treatment of choice in patients who can tolerate it.

21. What is an ERCP?

ERCP is an abbreviation for endoscopic retrograde cholangiopancreatography. ERCP is an endoscopy procedure with the objective of examining the bile duct or pancreatic duct.

The most common reason for performing an ERCP is when the healthcare provider suspects a stone in the bile duct. When patients have pain in the upper abdomen, in conjunction with enlargement of the bile duct on imaging such as an ultrasound or a CT scan, elevation in liver function tests on blood work, or jaundice, a bile duct stone is a strong possibility. An ERCP is also performed when there is suspicion of a blockage in the bile duct, either from benign inflammation or a tumor.

The pancreatic duct can also be examined by an ERCP, most commonly in patients with chronic pancreatitis with stones in the pancreatic duct. An ERCP may be useful in removing such stones, which helps in treating the pain from chronic pancreatitis in selected patients.

An ERCP is generally performed as an outpatient procedure, unless the patient is already admitted to the hospital. The procedure is performed with an anesthetic, either "conscious sedation" given through an

intravenous catheter, or general anesthesia administered by an anesthesiologist. Local anesthetic spray is
applied to the throat to numb the gag reflex. The test
generally takes between 30 and 90 minutes. Once the
patient is comfortably sedated, a flexible endoscope is
advanced into the mouth, through the esophagus and
stomach, and into the small intestine. The opening into
the bile duct and pancreatic duct (called the ampulla of
Vater) is identified in the small intestine. The gastroenterologist then passes a thin catheter under direct X-ray
guidance directly into the desired duct. Dye is injected
into the duct and X-ray images are taken. If a stone is
identified, it is removed by enlarging the opening to
the bile duct (called a sphincterotomy) and pulling the
stone out of the duct. The stone is left in the intestine
where it should pass without difficulty. If a blockage
is identified, a tissue sample may be obtained and sent
for analysis. A plastic or expandable metal tube called
a stent may also be left in the bile duct to allow bile to
drain from the liver and bypass the obstruction.

An ERCP is more invasive than a routine endoscopic
procedure and carries a higher risk of complications.
The most frequent complication is acute pancreatitis,
which occurs in about 5–10% of cases. In most cases,
pancreatitis following an ERCP requires admission
to the hospital for a few days. Rarely, the illness can
be severe or even life-threatening. Bleeding, infection,
and perforation of the intestine can also occur but are
less common. Rarely, blood transfusions or surgery are
necessary to manage these complications. An ERCP
is an advanced endoscopic procedure that is best performed by a physician experienced in this examination.

22. What are pancreatic cysts and how are they treated?

Pancreatic cysts are fluid-filled sac-like pouches located in or on the pancreas. Cysts can be either benign (noncancerous) or malignant (cancerous), but most are benign. In fact, many are pseudocysts—fluid-filled collections of scar tissue that result from multiple bouts of acute pancreatitis.

Small cysts (smaller than 2 cm) often do not cause enough pain or other symptoms to be noticeable. These cysts might be discovered during an abdominal scan (such as an ultrasound or MRI) for unrelated concerns. Larger cysts may cause abdominal pain. In addition, if a large cyst blocks the bile duct, it will cause bilirubin to back up into the blood stream, causing jaundice.

Your healthcare provider may suggest an endoscopic ultrasound, as it allows for closer inspection of the pancreas. During this procedure, the clinician is able to perform fine needle aspiration, a process in which a very thin needle is threaded through the endoscope and a small amount of fluid is drawn from the cyst. This fluid can be examined microscopically for the presence of cancerous cells.

Treatment varies depending on the size and type of cyst. Smaller, noncancerous, asymptomatic cysts may be left alone, although your healthcare provider may choose to monitor the cyst over time to check for growth or other changes. Larger cysts that are causing pain or blocking a duct may need to be drained, although there is a chance they will return with repeated bouts of pancreatitis. Drainage can be done via fine needle aspiration. Cancerous cysts should be surgically removed.

PART THREE

Exocrine Pancreatic Insufficiency

What is EPI (exocrine pancreatic insufficiency)?

What are digestive enzymes and what do they do?

Who is at risk for developing EPI?

More . . .

23. What is EPI (exocrine pancreatic insufficiency)?

Exocrine pancreatic insufficiency (EPI) is a condition in which the pancreas does not make enough digestive enzymes to enable adequate nutrition in the body. As stated, one of the major roles of the pancreas is to digest food. This involves breaking down the food to its more basic elements (proteins, carbohydrates, and fats), which allows the vitamins and nutrients to be taken into the body from the small intestine. When the pancreas does not produce enough enzymes to adequately digest food and allow the nutrients and vitamins to be absorbed, this results in EPI.

EPI is common in patients with chronic pancreatitis, so it is important that this condition is evaluated for in any patients with chronic pancreatitis.

24. What are digestive enzymes and what do they do?

The juice made by the pancreas to break down food is filled with enzymes. These pancreatic enzymes are critical to allow for proper digestion. Hundreds of specific types of enzymes are made in the pancreas, but they fall into three major categories: those which digest fat (lipases), those which digest carbohydrates (amylase), and those which digest protein (proteases and peptidases). In addition, a fluid called bicarbonate is made in the pancreas and serves to neutralize the stomach acid that mixes in with the food sent to the small intestine. It is important for food not to be too acidic for it to be properly digested in the small intestine.

Pancreatic enzymes are made in a part of the pancreas termed the acinar cell (hormones, in contrast, are made in the pancreatic islet cell). Bicarbonate is made in the pancreatic ductal cells. When pancreas enzymes are made, they are made in the non-active form. Upon stimulation from food in the stomach, a chemical signal (called **cholecystokinin** or CCK) is sent to the pancreas acinar cells, prompting release of the pancreatic enzymes into the small intestine. The enzymes are only "turned on" (activated) when they reach the small intestine. In their active form, these enzymes are then used to digest food that has come into the small intestine from the stomach.

In addition to the pancreas enzymes, the pancreas releases bicarbonate from its ductal cells when a signal is received from the stomach that there is food to digest. The chemical which tells the pancreas to release bicarbonate is called **secretin**. Both pancreatic enzymes and bicarbonate are essential to help with the proper digestion of food.

25. Who is at risk for developing EPI?

Patients with chronic damage to the pancreas are at risk for developing EPI. For example, most patients with chronic pancreatitis will have some degree of damage to the pancreas. While all patients with chronic pancreatitis may not necessarily have symptoms of EPI, usually there is at least some small degree of EPI present.

In addition, most patients with cystic fibrosis have some degree of EPI. This is because cystic fibrosis destroys the ductal cell of the pancreas, resulting in

Cholecystokinin

A hormone secreted by the small intestine that activates the gallbladder and stimulates the release of enzymes in the pancreas.

Secretin

A hormone produced in the small intestine that stimulates secretion of pancreatic juices.

varying degrees of pancreatic damage. Many patients with cystic fibrosis are born with a pancreas that does not function—as a result, they do not gain weight appropriately in their early years and often have significant diarrhea. The lack of weight gain and diarrhea is often what makes healthcare providers suspect cystic fibrosis as a cause in newborns and toddlers.

Finally, patients who have undergone pancreatic surgery are also at risk for developing EPI. Depending on the type and extent of the surgery, patients may require treatment for EPI. It is important to discuss the possibility of EPI with your surgeon following the procedure, as failure to gain weight, fatigue, and diarrhea could be related to untreated EPI.

26. What are the symptoms of EPI?

The classic symptom of EPI is foul-smelling diarrhea. Often, the diarrhea is streaked with fat, resulting in an "oil sheen" appearance in the toilet. The stool is often pale-appearing with streaks of yellow and can be difficult to flush. This type of stool, which is filled with undigested fat, is called steatorrhea. Classically, the pancreas must be severely damaged to experience significant steatorrhea. However, even patients with mild EPI can develop occasionally bouts of this type of stool.

Malabsorption

A condition in which the small intestine is not able to absorb nutrients and vitamins.

Because EPI results in the inability to properly digest food, the body often does not receive enough calories to maintain its weight. This is called **malabsorption**. Therefore, an inability to gain weight or even weight loss is commonly associated with EPI. Usually, patients with EPI simply cannot maintain their weight despite eating adequate amounts of food.

When food is not properly digested in the intestine, excess gas can occur. As a result, patients with EPI can develop excessive amounts of bloating, as well as belching and flatulence (passing gas from the rectum). Often, this gas is very unpleasant. Due to the bloating, abdominal pain usually centered in the abdomen can result.

Sometimes, patients with EPI do not have any obvious symptoms. However, when their blood is evaluated, they may have certain vitamin and mineral levels that are too low. The classic vitamin deficiencies (low levels in the blood) associated with EPI include lack of vitamins A, D, E, and K, as well as zinc. Vitamin A is important for vision, especially at night, so patients with vitamin A deficiency may have trouble seeing at night (a condition called "night blindness"). Vitamin D is important for strong bones, so commonly patients with low vitamin D levels will have thin bones (osteoporosis) or even easily suffer broken bones and fractures. Vitamin E is important for heart, skin, and bone health and vitamin K is important to help adequately clot the blood; patients with vitamin K deficiency can often develop easy bruising or bleeding. Finally, zinc is important for skin health, so rashes and sores can be more common in patients with this condition.

27. How is EPI diagnosed?

There are several different tests that can be used to diagnose EPI. The easiest test is to simply evaluate a patient's symptoms. For example, if a patient has known chronic pancreatitis and then develops steatorrhea, bloating, and weight loss, more than likely this is due to EPI. However, not every patient with EPI displays the classic symptoms. As a result, certain tests have been developed to help confirm the diagnosis.

Stool tests for fat: There are several different stool tests used to diagnose EPI. One test involves examining a single stool sample for fat, as excess fat on the stool is a classic symptom of EPI. Unfortunately, this test is not always accurate because one single sample may have varying amounts of fat. More commonly, a 72-hour stool collection is performed. This requires patients to eat a high amount of fat for three days (usually over 100 grams per day!) and collect all stool produced over those three days. The stool is then weighed in the lab and the fat content determined. If the level is over a certain limit, EPI can be diagnosed.

It is important to remember, though, that the presence of fat in the stool does not necessarily mean that a patient has EPI. There are several conditions (such as celiac disease) that can cause excess fat in the stool, so it is important to rule these conditions out before a diagnosis of EPI is made.

Stool elastase: Elastase is one of the enzymes that is made in the pancreas and is used to digest food in the small intestine. Normally, a certain amount of elastase is found in the stool. However, patients with EPI will not make as much elastase in their pancreas and thus will have less measurable elastase in the stool. Patients with a low stool elastase are considered to have EPI. While this test is widely available and easy to perform, some healthcare providers feel that it is somewhat inaccurate because it relies on only one stool sample.

Breath tests: There are several "breath tests" that can be used to evaluate for EPI. In these tests, patients are given a special meal or liquid to swallow that is broken down by pancreatic enzymes. The breakdown products of this special meal can be measured in the patient's breath by taking breath samples for approximately an hour after swallowing the meal. Depending on the amount of breakdown products in the breath, a diagnosis of EPI can sometimes be made. However, these tests are still in the development phase and currently are not widely used.

Pancreatic stimulation tests: While ideal for diagnosing EPI, pancreatic stimulation tests are expensive, invasive, and only available at specialized centers. The principle behind these tests is to stimulate the pancreas with a hormone and measure how many enzymes or how much bicarbonate is produced. Typically, a tube is placed into the small intestine just below where the pancreas empties its contents. Using an intravenous (IV) catheter, either CCK or secretin (CCK stimulates enzyme release and secretin stimulates bicarbonate release) is given in standard amounts. Next, the pancreas juice is collected over an hour and the amount of enzymes or bicarbonate is measured. If the levels are below the set standard, patients are diagnosed with EPI.

28. How is EPI treated?

EPI is treated in three different ways: 1) supplementing the diet with PERT, 2) limiting intake of foods which are not easily digested due to EPI, and 3) correcting vitamin deficiencies that result from EPI.

PERT is generally regarded as an effective treatment for EPI due to various conditions such as cystic fibrosis. Pancreatic enzymes are made from the ground up pancreases of pigs. The enzymes are purified and then packaged into capsules or pills of varying doses which are taken by mouth. Many different companies make enzymes, but essentially are all designed to perform the same function—to provide supplemental pancreatic enzymes when the pancreas is not able to work properly. By providing pancreatic enzymes in the small intestine at the time of eating, food can be digested properly. There are risks and side effects for PERT products and they may not be right for every patient. Please talk to your doctor about your medical condition and treatment choices.

In addition, fatty foods are the most difficult types of food to digest with EPI. By limiting the amount of fat in the diet, patients will have less malabsorption. In some patients, even stricter fat restriction is necessary. For patients who cannot tolerate any fat in their diet, an oily liquid containing medium-chain triglycerides, which are a type of fat that does not need pancreas enzymes to digest, can be supplemented in the diet.

Patients should also try to limit the amount of food they eat at each meal. Rather than having three large meals per day, patients often have less malabsorption when they "graze" throughout the day on small, frequent meals. Small, frequent meals are easier for the pancreas to digest, rather than large amounts of food all at once.

Finally, it is important to replace the vitamins which can be lost when patients have EPI. Most commonly, it is necessary to replace vitamin D. However, the other vitamins at risk to be low with EPI (vitamins A, E, and K) sometimes need to be replaced as well.

29. How do I take my enzymes?

No matter the type of pancreatic enzyme, you should talk with your physician about the dose of lipase units that is needed for each meal to adequately replace the enzymes needed for digestion. Always read and refer to the Medication Guide that comes with your PERT product before you start taking it for the first time and each time you get a refill. Each enzyme type is labeled to tell how many units of lipase are present in the medication. It is important, therefore, that if a patient has EPI, he or she gets enough units of lipase per day. Some patients may need slightly more or slightly less. Typically, patients can adjust the amount depending on their symptoms of malabsorption.

Enzymes should be taken at the time of each meal. While there is some controversy as to exactly when during the meal they should be taken, most healthcare providers would advise taking one enzyme just before the first bite of the meal, followed by taking the rest midway through the meal. If you forget to take your enzymes with a meal, you should wait until your next meal and take your scheduled number of capsules. Do not make up for missed doses.

PART FOUR

Pancreatic Cancer

What is pancreatic cancer?

How is pancreatic cancer diagnosed?

How is pancreatic cancer treated?

More . . .

30. What is pancreatic cancer?

Pancreatic cancer can be broken down into exocrine and endocrine types. Pancreatic cancer typically refers to pancreatic adenocarcinoma (also known as ductal adenocarcinoma), which involves the exocrine portion of the pancreas. Ductal adenocarcinomas arise mostly in the head of the gland (70%), but they also appear in the body (20%) and tail (10%). Adenocarcinomas of the pancreas account for more than 90% of all types of pancreatic cancers. Another type of pancreatic cancer is endocrine pancreatic cancer, also known as neuro-endocrine or islet cell cancer. These cancers usually arise in the body and tail of the pancreas and generally grow slowly, consequently having a better prognosis. Lymphomas and sarcomas also rarely occur in the pancreas. Lymphomas and sarcomas of the pancreas are treated the same as if they were located elsewhere in the body. Other unusual types of pancreatic malignancies include acinar cancers, adenosquamous variants of ductal adenocarcinoma, and solid and pseudopapillary cancer of the pancreas. The latter type is uncommon, but is most often seen in younger women and tends to have a significantly more favorable prognosis compared to ductal adenocarcinoma.

31. How is pancreatic cancer diagnosed?

Pancreatic cancer is diagnosed with good clinical insight and a variety of tests. Weight loss, decreased appetite, jaundice, and new diabetes should prompt suspicion for this disease. For many patients with jaundice, the typical starting tests are liver blood chemistries and an abdominal ultrasound. A high-quality computed tomography (CT) scan is probably the most useful test. A CT scan can show small tumors of the pancreas and whether the cancer has spread, for example, to the liver or the inner lining of the abdominal cavity (peritoneum). Dedicated pancreas CT scans (CT pancreas angiogram or pancreas protocol CT) provide very-fine definition of tumors and their relationship to important blood vessels that will help determine whether the cancer is operable. Most patients who are being considered for an operation and are likely to undergo surgery will have one of these scans performed. If you develop jaundice, an endoscopic retrograde cholangiopancreatogram (ERCP) allows the pancreas and common bile duct to be directly visualized. In addition, the latter test can allow placement of a stent, a plastic or metal tube that forces the bile duct open and permits bile flow and the relief of jaundice.

No specific blood tests have been established to diagnose pancreatic cancer at an early stage. However, Ca19–9, a substance found on the surface of and shed by adenocarcinoma cells, may be seen and measured in the bloodstream in the majority of patients with pancreatic cancer. Ca19–9 can serve as a tumor marker because to some extent, following Ca19–9 levels can track the course of the disease.

Sampling tissue from the pancreas itself (via a CT or ultrasound-guided biopsy) or taking scrapings (washings or brushings) from the lining of the pancreatic duct using an ERCP is usually needed to make the actual diagnosis of pancreatic cancer. Increasingly, the most useful test to diagnose pancreatic cancer is an endoscopic ultrasound (EUS). During an EUS, a small ultrasound probe is passed into the stomach or small bowel and the pancreatic tumor is visualized directly. A needle is passed into the tumor (fine needle aspirate) to secure a diagnosis. This procedure is performed under light anesthesia and usually a diagnosis is available within 1 to 2 days. One additional advantage of an EUS is that the relationship of the tumor to blood vessels can be identified and this may contribute to the determination of whether the tumor is operable. In patients with metastatic disease involving the liver or with ascites (fluid) in the abdominal cavity, taking a liver biopsy or sampling the ascites can confirm a diagnosis. Sometimes the diagnosis is strongly suspected before an operation, but is not confirmed until surgery is performed. This latter issue partly relates to the fact that pancreatic tumors can cause a very dense fibrosis/scarring-type reaction around the tumor, making it difficult to secure enough cells to confirm a diagnosis of cancer with a small needle.

32. How is pancreatic cancer treated?

Treatment for pancreatic cancer can be categorized as curative or palliative. Curative therapy means trying to get rid of the disease completely, and hence, there is hope for a long-term cure. This might be accomplished via chemotherapy, radiation, surgery, or a combination of these interventions.

Generally, all treatment for inoperable pancreatic cancer (i.e., both locally advanced and metastatic disease) is palliative and noncurative in intent. Palliative treatment is not useless; relief of symptoms and improving quality of life are major goals in treating patients with inoperable pancreatic cancer. When the cancer has spread, the goals of treatment are to affect the best control of the cancer for as long as possible, to extend life, to maximize your quality of life, and to minimize the negative impacts from the treatment.

Several other treatment options are available for patients with pancreatic cancer, one of which would be a clinical trial assessing new drugs, chemotherapy, or otherwise, that get in the way of certain cell functions. Several types of vaccines are also being developed as adjunctive treatments for pancreatic cancer. Another treatment strategy for pancreatic cancer is a "supportive-care" approach, which means that no active anticancer therapy is employed, but that all of the symptom-relieving measures are used (e.g., pain relief, relief of constipation, and drainage of ascites). Supportive-care treatments are included as part of the overall treatment plan for all patients with pancreatic cancer, but in patients with advancing end-stage disease, supportive-care treatments may be used exclusively.

Patient Perspective

Sue is a 61-year-old mother of three who had been in really good health until about three months ago. She has had diabetes for about ten years and always controlled her blood sugars well with a combination of healthy eating, daily exercise, and medications. However, in the last three months she began to notice that her blood sugar levels were much higher than normal, even though she had not changed anything about her lifestyle or medications. She was also happy because she had lost about 15 pounds during that time and really felt as though her exercise program was working well.

One week ago, however, she noticed that her urine was becoming darker—almost the color of tea—and her stools were becoming lighter. Yesterday, a friend told her that her eyes appeared "yellow" and she made an appointment to see her doctor. Her doctor sent her to the hospital for a CT scan to look at her pancreas. The scan showed a small mass in the head of the pancreas which appeared to be blocking her bile duct. Her doctor told Sue that she probably had pancreatic cancer.

Healthcare Provider Perspective

Sue had many of the signs and symptoms that can be associated with pancreatic cancer. For one, she had very well-controlled diabetes for several years and then suddenly, without explanation, her blood sugar levels became difficult to control. In about 60% of patients with pancreatic cancer, blood sugar levels can be abnormal up to 6 months before the diagnosis is made. In other words, patients with diabetes can have more difficulty controlling blood sugar, and patients without a previous diagnosis of diabetes can be found to have this disease before they are found to have cancer. This is because the cancer cells directly poison the cells in the pancreas that make insulin.

In addition, it is common for patients to have some weight loss prior to their diagnosis of cancer. It usually is only between 5–15 pounds, and often patients think that the weight loss may be due to a diet or exercise program.

One of the "classic" symptoms of pancreas cancer located in the head of the pancreas is the skin or eyes turning yellow—the medical term for this condition is jaundice. Most of the time patients do not have pain with the jaundice so the term providers use in these situations is "painless jaundice." Providers are taught to think of a diagnosis of pancreatic cancer when a patient is seen with painless jaundice—that is why the CT scan was performed. Other symptoms of jaundice

> *besides the yellow skin and eyes are dark-colored urine and light-colored stools. The CT scan shows a mass in the pancreas head. The mass is blocking the drainage tube of the liver—the bile duct—causing the bile not to flow well into the small intestine. When this happens, the patient will develop jaundice.*
>
> *Sue will be referred to a medical oncologist, a doctor who uses medications to treat cancer; a radiation oncologist, a doctor who uses radiation beams to treat cancer; and a surgical oncologist, a doctor who uses surgery to treat cancer, to discuss her treatment options. Depending on what stage of cancer she has, she can either undergo treatment with drugs and radiation, or have surgery. This will be a decision made between Sue and her treating doctors.*

33. What is chemotherapy and systemic therapy?

Chemotherapy is a medical drug treatment that is usually given intravenously, but occasionally orally, to treat cancers. Chemotherapy drugs are also called **cytotoxic** drugs, which means they are cell-destroying medications. Many different types of chemotherapeutic drugs exist that affect cancer cells in different ways by altering or interfering with differing parts of the cell cycle. Sometimes chemotherapy drugs are given alone and sometimes in a combination to try to achieve better control of the cancer. Systemic therapy is a broader term that encompasses both chemotherapy and newer "targeted"-type medications that have the potential to circulate in your body and address the disease at multiple sites. Systemic therapy can refer to both intravenous and oral medications.

Cytotoxic
Able to destroy cells.

Chemotherapy drugs affect rapidly dividing cells in the body, including cancer cells. The reason that side effects occur from chemotherapy is partly related to these effects on the cells that divide most rapidly (e.g., hair loss or irritation of the lining of the mouth or of the bowel [diarrhea]). In addition, some chemotherapy drugs have other side effects that are specific to that drug or class of drugs. Side effects of chemotherapy are also related to the dose and frequency of administration of the drugs as well as to characteristics of the patient (e.g., healthy, strong patients tolerate chemotherapy much better than sick, debilitated patients). Medication is sometimes required to minimize or counteract the side effects of chemotherapy.

34. What is biologic or targeted therapy?

Biologic therapy

New drug treatments that interfere with specific processes in cancer cell growth and development; also termed "targeted" therapy.

Mutated

Abnormal alteration in the structure of the DNA molecule (gene).

Targeted or **biologic therapy** refers to a new era of medications that are designed to more specifically focus on certain aspects of cancer cells over normal tissues. Many targeted therapies have been investigated as potential treatment options in pancreatic cancer. Thus far, however, this has been a relatively disappointing venture. Examples of targeted medications include drugs interfering with certain processes of cell growth and development. In most pancreatic cancers, the ras gene is known to be **mutated** (abnormal). This finding is exclusive to pancreatic cancer cells and not to normal pancreas tissue. Several drugs have been developed to target the ras pathway in cells, although the first generation of these drugs has not had any meaningful impact on pancreatic cancer. The next generation is in development and there is hope for greater effectiveness. Other examples of targeted medications include drugs that interfere with blood vessel growth and the development of tumors (e.g., antivascular agents). To date, antivascular agents have not been established to have usefulness in pancreatic cancer (they currently are effective on other cancers) but several **clinical trials** assessing newer antivascular agents are ongoing.

Clinical trial

Research studies designed to test new treatments on humans, including drugs.

35. What is radiation therapy?

Radiation therapy is X-ray treatment used to control and cure different types of cancer. Radiation is like surgery in that it is a localized type of treatment that affects small areas in the body, and it is different from chemotherapy or systemic therapy that circulates throughout the body. Radiation treatment is usually delivered daily, Monday to Friday. A treatment course, depending on the area being treated and on the size of the cancer and the treatment intent, can be anywhere from 5–10 treatments to 28–35 treatments. Very specific targets are marked out on your body, often using complicated CT scanning to determine the exact area to be treated. This process (called **simulation**) can take several hours. From there, medical physicists and the radiation oncologist plan the total dose of the radiation, the number of treatments, and the field size. Usually a couple of days before beginning radiation, you will undergo a "beam check" to ensure that the radiation prescription is exact and appropriate. Each daily radiation treatment takes approximately 10–15 minutes.

Simulation

Procedure that is part of the planning process for the administration of radiation therapy; involves X-rays or CT scans to identify the area to be treated and tattooing the skin to ensure correct positioning each day of treatment.

For pancreatic cancer, radiation treatment planning can be challenging because of the nearness of the stomach, the small bowel (duodenum), the spinal cord, the kidneys, and the like. Generally, after a treatment

Pancreatic Cancer

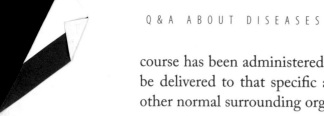
course has been administered, no further radiation can be delivered to that specific area because of effects to other normal surrounding organs and structures.

36. What is a Whipple operation and what side effects should I expect?

A Whipple operation is a major abdominal operation that is performed for cancers that are in the head of the pancreas, the duodenum, the ampulla (part of the duodenum), or the lower end of the common bile duct. It removes the head of the pancreas, part of the duodenum, and part of the bile duct and also involves reconnecting the bile duct to a different part of the small bowel, connecting a loop of bowel to the stomach, and reconnecting the pancreatic duct to the bowel. At the same time, many lymph nodes are taken out. This is an operation that takes several hours and is best performed by experienced surgeons who have specific expertise in this type of surgery.

When Whipple operations were first performed several decades ago, the complications and death rates were very high (25% or more). With years of experience, it is now much safer, and in good hands, the death rate is 2% to 3%. However, approximately 30% of the patients still develop problems after the surgery, but most of these are solved without long-term consequences.

Common complications of Whipple surgeries include delayed recovery of stomach movement, resulting in nausea, vomiting, and poor nutrition. This side effect can respond to medication and usually improves with time. Sometimes a surgeon can perform a modified type of Whipple surgery (pylorus-sparing procedure) to prevent this from happening. Wound infection and leakage of pancreatic juices (pancreatic fistula) are common, but generally get better with simple measures. Diabetes may occur or may be worsened as a result of surgery. Sometimes, the need for glucose-reducing drugs or insulin lessens over time; however, many patients will require treatment for diabetes. Many patients will have lost some weight before surgery, and most patients will lose approximately 10% to 15% of their total body weight in the 4– to 6–week period after surgery. The reasons for the weight loss are multiple and include more than just not eating for an extended period of time. With good dietary advice and nutritional supplements, weight loss can be reduced to some extent. Many patients will never regain all the weight that they lost and their new baseline weight is typically lower after such a surgery. Surgery can worsen postoperative weight loss because removal of even part of the pancreas results in loss of digestive enzymes that break down and digest food, which can lead to an inability to absorb important nutrients and consequently, EPI. Consequences of lack of enzymes include streatorrhea, gas, and weight loss.

37. What is a pancreatectomy and what are the associated complications?

A pancreatectomy is surgical removal of the pancreas, which can be categorized as complete (total removal of pancreas and parts of surrounding organs), central (removal of the mid portion of the pancreas), or distal (removal of the mid and tail portions of the pancreas, the spleen, and sometimes part of the stomach).

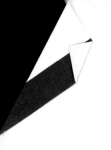

Many of the complications following a pancreatectomy are similar to those following a Whipple procedure, such as nausea, vomiting, abdominal pain, diarrhea, cramping, risk of wound infection, and risk of pancreatic fistula. Patients experiencing some form of partial pancreatectomy may experience diabetes or exocrine pancreatic insufficiency (EPI). However, patients who undergo complete pancreatectomy are guaranteed these outcomes. Those patients, therefore, will require lifelong supplemental insulin injections and PERT.

One treatment option for avoiding post-pancreatectomy diabetes is via total pancreatectomy with autoislet cell transplant (TPIAT). TPIAT is an uncommon, but often effective, way of treating pain symptoms from chronic or recurrent acute pancreatitis.

TPIAT is a technique that is used to prevent development of diabetes in patients who undergo complete removal of their pancreas. The technique works as follows: When a patient has his or her pancreas completely removed, the pancreas is brought to a special laboratory. In the laboratory, the pancreas is broken down with a variety of different chemicals so just the parts of the pancreas (the islet cells) which make insulin and the other important hormones in the pancreas are left over. The islet cells are then put back into the liver of the patient who underwent the pancreatectomy. The term "auto" (short for **autologous**) describes the fact that the islet cells that are put into the liver are from the same patient. The term "allo" (short for **allogeneic**) refers to a transplant in which organs and tissues are taken from one patient and placed into another patient. Ideally, the islet cells start to grow in the liver and start producing the chemicals, like insulin, which are important to maintain the correct blood sugar levels. It is

Autologous

Obtained from the same organism or individual.

Allogeneic

Derived from individuals who are genetically unlike but are of the same species.

hoped that the islet cells in the liver will grow to the point where the patient does not become a diabetic.

However, there are some drawbacks to this procedure. Probably the biggest drawback is that it is very difficult to break down the pancreas and harvest the islet cells. As a result, only a few big hospitals in the world perform this procedure. Also, the islet cells do not always work effectively, even if they are put into the liver correctly, and this can cause people to become diabetic anyway. Finally, it is often very difficult to choose which patients will benefit the most from TPIAT because in many patients, removing the entire pancreas does not lead to relief of pain.

Therefore, it is very important to have a discussion with your healthcare providers about the advantages and disadvantages of such a major surgery before going forward. It is also important to visit a hospital which performs the procedure regularly.

Another procedure that is sometimes considered is a pancreas allo (short for allogeneic) transplant, which is a transplant in which a pancreas from one patient is placed into someone else. The pancreas that is transplanted is acquired after a patient dies and he/she or a family member has expressed an interest in **organ donation**.

Soon after the patient wishing to donate his/her pancreas dies, the pancreas is removed by a surgical team in the hospital and brought to the waiting patient. The pancreas is then placed into the new patient in a complicated operation. Once the pancreas has been placed into the new patient, that patient must take medications, called **immunosuppressants**, for the rest of his or her life to make sure the pancreas works properly.

Organ donation

Surgical removal and transplantation of organs from a donor to a recipient.

Immuno-suppressants

Drugs that are used to suppress or lower the body's immune function.

Most often, pancreas transplants are performed to help prevent complications of diabetes. Therefore, most patients who receive a pancreas transplant have difficult-to-control diabetes. Pancreas transplants are all performed in people who have had to have their pancreas removed for various reasons.

Because there are many more people who need pancreas transplants than there are pancreases available, patients who are eligible for a transplant must be registered on a transplant list. The transplant list is maintained by the hospital at which the transplant will be performed. Patients on the transplant list usually carry a beeper or phone for several months until they are called to come receive their transplant. A goal of the medical community is to increase the number of pancreases available for transplant.

38. Can I live without a pancreas?

Believe it or not, patients can live happy, productive lives without a pancreas! However, immediately following a pancreatectomy, patients will develop two serious medical issues: the inability to make pancreas enzymes and diabetes. If those patients do not take pancreas enzyme supplements, they will develop severe malabsorption and malnutrition. This is a condition that cannot be fixed and will require those patients to stay on pancreatic enzymes for their entire life. The diabetes will require patients to use insulin injections for the rest of their lives.

Many patients ask us why they cannot simply have their pancreas removed, especially if they are struggling with the pain from chronic pancreatitis. The reason removing the whole pancreas is not done very often is because of these two side effects (diabetes and malabsorption). It is often thought that having these two side effects from removing the pancreas is worse than keeping the pancreas in place.

A word of caution to patients is that if it has been recommended that you have a complete pancreatectomy, make sure you discuss these side effects with your healthcare provider before proceeding with the surgery.

Pancreatic Cancer

PART FIVE

Related Conditions

What is cystic fibrosis?

How is cystic fibrosis related to diseases of
the pancreas?

Are there other disorders related to
pancreas disease?

More . . .

39. What is cystic fibrosis?

Cystic fibrosis is an inherited disease of mucus and sweat glands that can cause malabsorption. It can affect the lungs, pancreas, liver, intestines, and sinuses. Normally, mucus is watery and keeps linings of organs moist to prevent infection. In cystic fibrosis, an abnormal **gene** causes mucus to become sticky and thick. When this problem is mostly focused in the lungs, patients can develop difficulty breathing with frequent lung infections like pneumonia. Eventually, the infections in the lung can become so severe that patients can no longer breathe well.

A great deal of research is currently being performed to try to develop drugs which will improve how the mucous and sweat glands work in patients with cystic fibrosis.

Gene

A hereditary unit located on a chromosome that contains a sequence of DNA.

40. How is cystic fibrosis related to diseases of the pancreas?

Because cystic fibrosis causes the body's mucus to become sticky and thick, this mucus can block tubes or ducts in the pancreas. Digestive enzymes produced in the pancreas cannot reach the small bowel and cannot absorb fats and proteins fully.

In some patients with severe cystic fibrosis, the pancreas is destroyed while still **in utero** (inside the mother) and the baby is born with the inability to make pancreatic enzymes. As a result, the baby does not grow well and becomes malnourished. The malnutrition can be treated, however, with pancreatic enzymes.

In utero

In the uterus (before birth).

Increasingly, doctors are finding that patients can have cystic fibrosis of the pancreas even if they do not have any lung disease. This is because cystic fibrosis can affect each organ differently. In the pancreas, some patients can have occasional bouts of acute pancreatitis caused by cystic fibrosis. In others, patients can develop painful chronic pancreatitis. How the pancreas is affected in each person really depends on how altered the cystic fibrosis gene is in that person.

41. Are there other disorders related to pancreas disease?

There are a few other conditions that are related to pancreatic disease. Celiac disease, which is a common, inherited allergy to a part of wheat, barley, and oats can cause the pancreas not to work effectively in some patients. The part of wheat, barley, and oats which people with celiac disease react to is called **gluten**. These patients are treated with pancreatic enzymes and told to avoid gluten products in their diet.

Certain cancers, not starting in the pancreas, can move to the pancreas when they spread (**metastasize**) in the body. Some of the more common cancers which move to the pancreas when they spread are a type of skin cancer called melanoma, breast cancer, and lung cancer.

Gluten

A mixture of proteins found in cereal grains, especially wheat.

Metastasize

Growing or spreading to other sites in the body.

PART SIX

Nutrition and Pancreatic Disease

What is malabsorption and how is it different from malnutrition?

How do I know if I am not absorbing all of my nutrients and am becoming malnourished?

What are the long-term effects of malabsorption?

More . . .

42. What is malabsorption and how is it different from malnutrition?

Malabsorption and malnutrition are not the same condition. Malabsorption refers to a condition in which food is swallowed, but cannot be taken into the body appropriately. For example, some patients with chronic pancreatitis can eat a large amount of food. However, when that food reaches the intestine, there are not enough pancreas enzymes to help break down the food appropriately. As a result, the food that is taken in is not used properly and the body does not get the nutritional benefit of the food.

There are many causes of malabsorption—basically, most problems arising along the gastrointestinal system can lead to problems with malabsorption. Problems in the intestine, pancreas, and liver can all lead to malabsorption. **Table 3** lists some common causes of malabsorption.

Malnutrition refers to a condition in which the body does not have enough of the basic building blocks to function properly. There are two main reasons why a patient can become malnourished—either they are not taking in enough (or are taking in the wrong kinds of) food, or the body is not able to adequately absorb (malabsorption) the food that is being taken into the body. In other words, malabsorption is one of the causes of malnutrition.

Table 3   Common Causes of Malabsorption

Intestinal Disease
Celiac disease, Crohn's disease, lactose intolerance
Pancreatic Disease
Chronic pancreatitis
Exocrine pancreatic insufficiency (EPI)
Liver Disease
Tumors of the liver and bile ducts
Gallbladder removal

43. How do I know if I am not absorbing all of my nutrients and am becoming malnourished?

One of the most common signs that patients are mal-absorbing their food is weight loss. Because the body cannot take what it needs from the food being eaten, it is almost as if the body is not getting any food at all! Therefore, almost all patients who have malabsorption will have weight loss, although weight loss can occur for many other reasons besides malabsorption.

Another common symptom of malabsorption is diarrhea. Usually patients with malabsorption will have at least some loose stools. Often the stools are oily, meaning that there is malabsorbed fat in the stool. Other symptoms of malabsorption can be abdominal pain, nausea, vomiting, and a decrease in energy level.

The symptoms of being malnourished can be difficult to pin down because there are many different nutrients that are related to malnutrition in a patient. Generally, patients who are malnourished may have decreased energy levels and weight loss and may also experience skin rashes, blurry vision, nausea, and vomiting. However, it is very important to speak to your healthcare provider about your specific symptoms and questions, as this will determine what type of nutritional testing needs to be performed.

44. What are the long-term effects of malabsorption?

Most patients with longstanding malabsorption will eventually develop malnutrition if their condition is not recognized. Depending on the type of nutrients that are being malabsorbed, there could be permanent problems that develop. For example, many patients with chronic pancreatitis develop decreased levels of vitamin D. Decreased vitamin D levels can lead to bone loss, which can cause increased risk of thin bones (osteroporosis) and fractures. It is important, therefore, that this problem be evaluated and treated before thin bones develop. Many times, early detection of nutritional deficiencies can prevent further harm to the body, making it very important that patients at risk for malabsorption be tested.

Patient Perspective

Sally is 45 years old and has been very healthy for most of her life. However, about six months ago, she began to develop diarrhea. At first, she had 4–5 loose stools every day. The stools were watery and "oily" and were difficult to flush down the toilet. In the last month, she has had more stools—up to about 10 per day—and sometimes she even has to wake up in the middle of night to have a bowel movement. She has no pain, but has lost 30 pounds in the last three months. She is constantly hungry and feels like she cannot get enough to eat.

She went to her doctor's office and had a test of her stool, which showed a large amount of fat present. She then underwent a CT scan which showed her pancreas to be scarred and small, and she was diagnosed with chronic pancreatitis. She has no risk factors for chronic pancreatitis, but her father died in his 30s in a car accident and had often complained of indigestion.

Heathcare Provider Perspective

Sally has severe malabsorption related to her chronic pancreatitis. The reason for this is that her pancreas is not making enough enzymes to help her properly digest her food. This condition is called exocrine pancreatic insufficiency (EPI). Although she is eating a large amount of food, not all of it is being effectively used by her body and as a result, she is not getting enough nutrients.

She very likely has chronic pancreatitis that was passed on by her father—called hereditary pancreatitis. Although we cannot test her father for certain, it is likely that he too had pancreatitis, given he often complained about indigestion. One way to find out if Sally has hereditary pancreatitis would be to perform a blood test and check for genes which could have caused her pancreatitis.

Sally's treatment will be to limit the amount of fat in her diet and take pancreatic enzyme supplements. Pancreatic enzyme supplements should help to improve her weight loss by allowing her to appropriately digest her food. Once she is started on enzymes, it would be expected that she would gain back much of the weight that she lost.

It would also be important to check her for vitamin deficiencies, like low vitamin A and D levels, and replace these if they are low. Pancreatic enzymes may help in vitamin absorption. Often patients with EPI also require some vitamin supplements.

45. What foods and beverages should I eat or avoid if I have pancreatitis?

Patients often wonder what foods or beverages they should eat or avoid if they have been diagnosed with pancreatitis. In general, it is most beneficial to avoid rich, fatty foods, which stimulate the pancreas. While any type of food can make the pancreas active, it is the very fatty foods that patients are encouraged to avoid. This is not to say that patients with pancreatic disease should never eat fatty foods; but these should generally be kept in moderation. Patients on PERT therapy should take their medication with food, especially with fatty food, to allow for proper digestion. Drinks should also be monitored closely for fat content—especially some of the weight-gaining drinks that have a high amount of calories. **Table 4** lists foods that are best avoided if you have pancreatitis.

It is also important not to eat too much at one sitting. This is because putting a large amount of food in the stomach can cause the pancreas to work very hard, which can lead to having more pain. Try to limit your diet to small, frequent meals. In other words, rather than having three large meals per day, it may be best to have 7–8 smaller meals scattered throughout the day.

Table 4   Types of Food to Avoid with Pancreatitis

Deep fried foods (i.e., onion rings, fried dough)
Fatty meats (i.e., use only lean ground beef)
Buttery foods
Milk shakes
High calorie protein shakes

Of course, each individual patient is different and what might be appropriate for one patient may not be the best for another. A general rule of thumb is that if you eat something and develop pancreatic pain, it is best to avoid that same food in the future!

PART SEVEN

Living with Pancreatic Disease

How do I maximize visits with my
healthcare provider?

Do I need to make any changes to my lifestyle?

Can I continue to exercise if I have a disease
of the pancreas?

More . . .

46. How do I maximize visits with my healthcare provider?

It is very important to try to understand as much as possible about your condition prior to a visit with your healthcare provider. Great resources are the websites listed at the end of this book. You can also read about the different diseases that can affect the pancreas— acute pancreatitis, chronic pancreatitis, pancreatic cancer, and so forth. Most people do not know a great deal about the pancreas, so having at least a little bit of knowledge before the appointment can really help you to ask important questions about your disease.

It is very helpful for your healthcare provider to have an up-to-date and accurate list at your appointment of all medications you take. In addition, a thorough knowledge of your medical history, as well as the treatments and evaluations that have been tried before, can usually be very helpful.

Virtually all decisions regarding how to treat your pancreatic disease will rely on X-rays that have been performed before the appointment. Usually, these X-rays take the form of a CT scan or an MRI scan. These X-rays are usually stored on CDs and it is critical for your provider to have these when you are seen for your appointment. Often, it only takes a phone call to your healthcare provider's office to make sure the CD is available. However, if not, you should make sure to bring a copy with you to the appointment. Copies can usually be picked up free of charge at the facility where you had your X-rays taken.

It is very important to arrive between 20–30 minutes prior to the first appointment. The healthcare provider's office may have paperwork to fill out and you really want to maximize the amount of time you have with your healthcare provider.

Sometimes it is possible to coordinate many of your appointments on the same day. For example, if you know that you are going to need a CT scan performed, you can call ahead and ask your healthcare provider to coordinate these appointments on the same day. This can be very helpful and efficient, especially if you live far away.

If there is no medical reason not to, it is sometimes reasonable to try to come to the appointment not having eaten or drunk since midnight the night before the appointment. This can aid your healthcare provider if, for example, there are lab tests that need to be performed that require fasting, or if your healthcare provider would like to schedule an X-ray test or perhaps have you undergo a procedure that same day. Of course, this is not a requirement and should not be undertaken if there is a medical reason not to fast. You can also call your healthcare provider's office a few days ahead of the appointment to see if fasting would be appropriate.

47. Do I need to make any changes to my lifestyle?

Positive lifestyle changes can often help to improve symptoms of any digestive disease, even diseases of the pancreas. Stress reduction can be helpful. Avoiding overeating, fatty and fried foods, alcohol (if you have pancreatitis), smoking, and caffeine can also be beneficial. Although it may sound old-fashioned, getting a good night's sleep and resting when you are fatigued are helpful as well. Regular exercise and relaxation-targeted activities such as yoga can be helpful. If you have developed diabetes and/or malabsorption, you will need to incorporate taking medication such as insulin or pancreas enzymes into your lifestyle.

48. Can I continue to exercise if I have a disease of the pancreas?

Regular exercise, along with eating a healthy diet, helps promote a long and healthy life. People with a disease of the pancreas are encouraged to engage in routine exercise, taking a few precautions. If you are feeling particularly fatigued, it may be best not to push yourself too much during a workout. Although regular exercise is beneficial in the long term, at times it can do harm in the short term. So, exercise to stay fit, but only if you are fit enough to exercise. It is best to consult with your healthcare provider before starting an exercise regimen. Together, you two can decide what type of exercise is best for you.

49. How does pancreatic disease affect pregnancy?

While uncommon, pancreatic disease can develop during pregnancy. Acute pancreatitis is the most common reason why the pancreas can become ill during pregnancy. It is estimated that acute pancreatitis occurs in about 1 out of every 10,000 pregnancies. Most of the time, acute pancreatitis in pregnancy is caused by gallstone disease. It is thought that with the weight and hormonal changes caused by pregnancy, gallstones are more likely to form and thus travel down the common bile duct to obstruct the pancreas duct.

The treatment of acute pancreatitis in pregnancy is similar to that of non-pregnant patients with some exceptions. Resting the digestive tract by not eating, pain control, and aggressive fluids given through an IV line are essential. Typically, if the reason is gallstone pancreatitis, removal of the gallbladder is postponed until after pregnancy. However, if waiting until the end of pregnancy is not possible, surgical removal of the gallbladder can generally be performed safely.

Fortunately, it is very rare for either the mother or baby to die from acute pancreatitis. However, about 20% of the time, labor starts early. It is very important, therefore, that pregnant patients proceed as soon as possible to the emergency room for evaluation should they develop any abnormal abdominal pain symptoms.

While there are few published reports focusing on chronic pancreatitis and pregnancy, our experience has been that patients who become pregnant and have chronic pancreatitis generally do very well. It is important for patients with chronic pancreatitis to follow closely with their healthcare provider during pregnancy to make sure no complications develop. For those patients who are pregnant or considering becoming pregnant, talk with you doctor before starting to take any PERT product, because it is not known if they will harm an unborn baby.

50. Where can I find a support group?

There are many resources available for people diagnosed with a disease of the pancreas. For example, the organization Pancreatica.org lists a wealth of information about pancreatic cancer and maintains a large database on relevant clinical trials. A list of useful organizations and their contact information is shown in **Table 5**. In addition, your healthcare provider may be familiar with resources and support groups in your area.

Table 5   Resources on Pancreas Disease

Name of Organization	Web site	Phone
Association of Online Cancer Resources	http://www.acor.org	
Digestive Disease National Coalition	http://www.ddnc.org	1-202-544-7497
National Pancreas Foundation	http://pancreasfoundation.org	1-866-726-2737
Pancreatic Cancer Action Network	http://www.panCAN.org	1-877-272-6226
Pancreatic Cancer Alliance	http://www.pancreaticalliance.org	
Pancreatic Disease Center	http://www.ucpancreas.org	
Pancreatica	http://www.pancreatica.org	1-800-525-3777
The Pancreatitis Association, Inc	http://www.pancassociation.org	1-317-340-7513
The Pancreatitis Place	http://www.thepancreatitisplace.org	1-434-409-7162

Glossary

Abdominal X-ray: A radiologic examination that provides an image of structures and organs in the abdomen—helpful in detecting a bowel obstruction or perforation.

Abscess: A walled-off collection of pus; in Crohn's disease, an abscess is most commonly found around the anus or rectum, but can occur anywhere in the body.

Absorption: The process of taking nutrients into the tissues.

Acute cholecystitis: An inflammation of the gallbladder, most often due to gallstones, marked by severe abdominal pain and may be accompanied by fever.

Allogeneic: Derived from individuals who are genetically unlike but are of the same species.

Ampulla of Vater: Location of the major drainage from the pancreatic duct into the small intestine.

Amylases: Pancreatic enzymes that digest starches.

Anus: The outside opening of the rectum.

Autodigestion: The process by which prematurely activated pancreatic enzymes digest the pancreas, leading to acute pancreatitis.

Autologous: Obtained from the same organism or individual.

Barium enema: A radiologic examination of the rectum and colon performed by instilling barium through the rectum and taking X-rays as it travels through the colon; an excellent test to detect strictures, inflammation, and fistulas in the colon.

Bile: Thick, green fluid produced by the liver which plays an important role in the digestion of fats. Bile is made by the liver, stored by the gallbladder, and released into the bile duct and small intestine after meals.

Bile duct: A channel through which bile flows from the liver to the intestines.

Bilirubin: Product of the breakdown of hemoglobin, which can be measured to evaluate the liver and gallbladder.

Biologic therapy: New drug treatments that interfere with specific processes in cancer cell growth and development; also termed "targeted" therapy.

Biopsy: Usually performed during an endoscopy, a small piece of mucosa (inside lining of the intestine) is removed and examined under a microscope; an excellent test to characterize types of inflammation and detect dysplasia and cancer.

Bowel: Another name for intestine; that is, small intestine means the same as small bowel.

Cecum: The first part of the large intestine; a pouch-like area into which the ileum opens.

Cholangitis: Infection of the bile ducts; can occur in primary sclerosing cholangitis (PSC).

Cholecystectomy: Surgical removal of the gallbladder. The preferred technique is called laparoscopic cholecystectomy. The surgeon removes the gallbladder by inserting instruments into four small incisions in the abdominal wall. The traditional technique, sometimes called "open cholecystectomy," requires a larger incision in the right upper abdomen. Because of this larger scar, the pain after surgery and overall recovery time last longer with open cholecystectomy.

Cholecystokinin: A hormone secreted by the small intestine that activates the gallbladder and stimulates the release of enzymes in the pancreas.

Cholecystostomy: Drainage tube placed through the skin directly into the gallbladder. This tube is placed to treat infection of the gallbladder called acute cholecystitis. Cholecystotomy tubes are inserted when patients are too ill to withstand surgery to remove the gallbladder.

Chronic: Usually refers to a disease that develops slowly and lasts for a long time.

Cirrhosis: Formation of permanent scar tissue in the liver due to a chronic condition.

Clinical trial: Research studies designed to test new treatments on humans, including drugs.

Colitis: inflammation of the colon; can be due to Crohn's disease, ulcerative colitis, or other diseases.

Colon: The part of the large intestine that processes waste.

Colonoscopy: An endoscopic procedure in which a small, thin, flexible lighted tube with a camera on the end is passed through the rectum into the colon and, at times, into the ileum; an excellent test to detect inflammation and strictures in the rectum, colon, and ileum, and one that allows for a biopsy to be taken.

Common bile duct: Tube which connects the liver and gallbladder to the duodenum and drains bile into the small intestine.

Corticosteroid: A type of medication given to reduce inflammation. Corticosteroids come in oral and topical forms.

Cytotoxic: Able to destroy cells.

Duodenum: The first part of the small intestine, starting at the end of the stomach.

Endocrine: Referring to the hormone-producing function of the pancreas.

Enterokinase: A chemical within the small intestine which allows the pancreas enzymes to be unwrapped and begin digesting food.

Esophagus: Tube that carries food from the mouth to the stomach.

Exocrine: Referring to the digestion function of the pancreas.

Exocrine pancreatic insufficiency (EPI): When the pancreas fails to produce enough digestive enzymes to support adequate nutrient absorption.

Extracorporeal shock wave lithotripsy (ESWL): Noninvasive technique using high-energy sound waves to break up gallstones. Because this procedure is most frequently performed to break up kidney stones, it is generally performed by a urologist.

Fistula: A tunnel connecting two structures that are not normally connected; examples include a fistula between the rectum and vagina (rectovaginal fistula) or the colon and bladder (colovesicular fistula).

Gallbladder: Pouch connected to the bile ducts that stores bile, which is released with eating to aid in digestion.

Gallstones: Stones that form in the gallbladder.

Gastrocolic reflex: A reflex in which the act of eating or food entering the stomach stimulates movement in the colon and/or small intestine.

Gastroenterologist: A physician who specializes in diseases of the gastrointestinal tract, liver, and pancreas.

Gastrointestinal tract: The digestive tube that starts at the mouth and ends at the anus.

Gene: A hereditary unit located on a chromosome that contains a sequence of DNA.

Glucagon: A hormone made by the pancreas which also helps to control blood sugar.

Gluten: A mixture of proteins found in cereal grains, especially wheat.

Heterozygote: An individual who has two different forms of a particular gene (one normal, the other either dominant or recessive).

Ileum: Lowest section of the small intestine.

Immunosuppressants: Drugs that are used to suppress or lower the body's immune function.

In utero: In the uterus (before birth).

Inflammation: A process characterized by swelling, warmth, redness, and/or tenderness; can occur in any organ.

Insulin: a hormone made by the pancreas which helps to turn food into energy.

Islet cells: The microscopic parts of the pancreas which make hormones.

Jaundice: Yellowing of the skin due to buildup of bile. The most common causes of jaundice are hepatitis (infection of the liver), and blockage of the outflow of bile from the liver into the intestine from either a stone in the bile duct or a tumor.

Jejunum: The middle section of the small intestine; between the duodenum and ileum.

Large intestine: Also called colon; processes and stores waste.

Lipases: Pancreatic enzymes that digest fat.

Malabsorption: A condition in which the small intestine is not able to absorb nutrients and vitamins.

Metastasize: Growing or spreading to other sites in the body.

Motility system: The spontaneous contractions that move food through the gastrointestinal tract.

Mucosa: The innermost lining of the intestines.

Mutated: Abnormal alteration in the structure of the DNA molecule (gene).

Nasogastric tube: A long, flexible tube that is passed through the nose into the stomach and is used to suction out the stomach in the setting of a bowel obstruction or sometimes after an operation.

Obstruction: A blockage of the small intestine or colon.

Oncologist: A physician whose area of expertise is diagnosis and treatment of tumors.

Organ donation: Surgical removal and transplantation of organs from a donor to a recipient.

Pancreatic cyst: a fluid-filled cavity in the pancreas that can sometimes cause acute pancreatitis if it is blocking the pancreatic duct.

Pancreatic ducts: Drainage tubes of the pancreas.

Perforation: A rupture or abnormal opening of the intestine that allows intestinal contents to escape into the abdominal cavity.

Pharynx: Structure in the throat that connects directly with the beginning of the intestinal tract or esophagus.

Proteases: Pancreatic enzymes that digest protein.

Pseudocyst: Fluid-filled collection of tissue in or adjacent to the pancreas. Pseudocysts form as a consequence of either acute or chronic pancreatitis and can cause problems when they become infected or grow so large that they block digestion of nutrients or drainage of pancreas juice.

Rapid intestinal transit: An increase in propulsion in the colon, such that the colon contracts more intensely than normal and food passes through more quickly.

Rectum: Last part of colon where stool is stored until it leaves the digestive tract.

Salivary gland: Glands in the mouth that produce material that aid in the breakdown of food.

Secretin: A hormone produced in the small intestine that stimulates secretion of pancreatic juices.

Sedation: Also called conscious sedation, or moderate sedation; sedation is a form of moderate anesthesia in which the patient is given medication to induce a state of relaxation. Patients under sedation are sleepy and are less likely to feel discomfort.

Simulation: Procedure that is part of the planning process for the administration of radiation therapy; involves X-rays or CT scans to identify the area to be treated and tattooing the skin to ensure correct positioning each day of treatment.

Sjögren's syndrome: A disorder of the immune system that affects the body's production of tears and saliva.

Small intestine: The small bowel is made up of the duodenum, jejunum, and ileum. Anatomically, it is found after the stomach and before the colon and is responsible for digestion and absorption of nutrients.

Sphincterotomy: A surgical procedure to open a muscle sphincter wide enough for gallstones to pass through.

Steatorrhea: The presence of excess fat in the stool.

Stricture: A narrowed area of intestine usually caused by scar tissue.

Tumor: An abnormal growth of tissue; can be benign or malignant.

Ultrasound: A radiologic study that uses sound waves to examine abdominal and pelvic organs; commonly used to look for gallstones and obstruction of the bile duct.

Uncinate: the part of the pancreas that wraps up and under the "head" of the pancreas and sometimes circles the small intestine.

Upper endoscopy: A procedure in which a small, thin, flexible, lighted tube with a camera on the end is passed through the mouth into the esophagus, stomach, and duodenum; an excellent test to detect inflammation and strictures in the upper gastrointestinal tract that allows a biopsy to be taken.

Upper GI series/upper GI series with small bowel follow-through (SBFT): A radiologic examination of the esophagus, stomach, duodenum, and small bowel. The patient drinks a thick, white liquid shake of barium, and then the barium is tracked by taking X-rays as it travels through the gastrointestinal tract. This is an excellent test to detect strictures, fistulas, and inflammation in the stomach and small bowel.

Villi: Finger-like projections lining the small intestine; involved in the digestion and absorption of food and nutrients.

INDEX

Index

Common bile duct, 10
Computed tomography (CT) scan, 6, 7
  high quality, 56–57
  for jaundice, 61
Conscious sedation. *See* Sedation
Corticosteroids, 35
Crohn's disease, 6
CT scan. *See* Computed tomography scan
Curative therapy, 58
Cystic fibrosis, 27, 47–48, 72
  and diseases of pancreas, 72–73
Cysts, pancreatic, 11-12, 21, 42
Cytotoxic drugs, 61–62

D

Digestion of food, 3–6
Digestive enzymes, 46–47, 72
Digestive system, 2–3, 2*f*
  test for, 6–10
Ductal adenocarcinomas. *See* Pancreatic
  adenocarcinoma
Duodenum, 4
Dye, 20, 41

E

Elastase, 50–51
Endocrine, 10
Endocrine pancreatic cancer, 56
Endoscopic retrograde cholangiopan-
    creatography (ERCP), 9, 20–23,
    29–30, 40–41, 57
Endoscopic ultrasound (EUS), 9–10, 57–58
  for diagnosing chronic pancreatitis, 29
Endoscopy, 20, 22, 40
  capsule, 9
  upper, 7, 9
Enteroclysis, 7
Enterokinase, 16
Enteroscopy, 8
Enzymes, 53
  digestive, 46–47
  pancreatic, 16, 27, 30, 46-47, 51-52, 68,
    72-73
EPI. *See* Exocrine pancreatic insufficiency
ERCP. *See* Endoscopic retrograde cholan-
  giopancreatography
Esophagus, 4
EUS. *See* Endoscopic ultrasound
Exocrine, 10
Exocrine pancreatic insufficiency (EPI),
    31, 79
  definition of, 46

diagnosis of, 49–51
risk for developing, 47–48
symptom of, 48–49
treatment for, 51–53
Extracorporeal shock wave lithotripsy
    (ESWL), 30, 39–40

F

Fat, stool tests for, 50
Fistula, 6
Food, digestion of, 3–6

G

Gallbladder, 3, 9–10, 11*f*, 18–19, 36
  disease, 23
  sludge, 37
Gallstones, 7, 18, 19
  pancreatitis, 87
  risk factor for, 37
  treatment for, 37–40
Gastrocolic reflex, 5–6
Gastroenterologist, 13
Gastrointestinal tract, 3
Gene, 72
Glucagon, 10, 11
Gluten, 73

H

Hereditary pancreatitis, 35–36, 79
Heterozygote, 27
Hormones, 3
Human digestive system, 2–3, 2*f*
Hydrases, 46

I

IgG4 level, 35
Ileum, 5
Immunosuppressants, 67
Inflammation, 6
Insulin, 10
Intravenous (IV) catheter, 51
In utero, 72
Islet cell cancer. *See* Endocrine pancreatic
    cancer
Islet cells, 10, 66–67

J

Jaundice, 34, 40, 42, 56-57
symptoms of, 61–62
Jejunum, 4

Index